CLINICAL TUBERCULOSIS

A PRACTICAL HANDBOOK

Edited by

Peter D O Davies, MA, DM, FRCP
Professor and Consultant Physician,
Liverpool Heart and Chest Hospital, UK

Ajit Lalvani, MA, DM, FRCP, FSB, FMedSci
Chair of Infectious Diseases, Director, Tuberculosis Research Centre,
National Heart and Lung Institute, Imperial College London, UK

Muhunthan Thillai, BA, MBBS, MRCP, PhD
Consultant Chest Physician, Interstitial Lung Disease Unit,
Papworth and Cambridge University Hospitals, UK

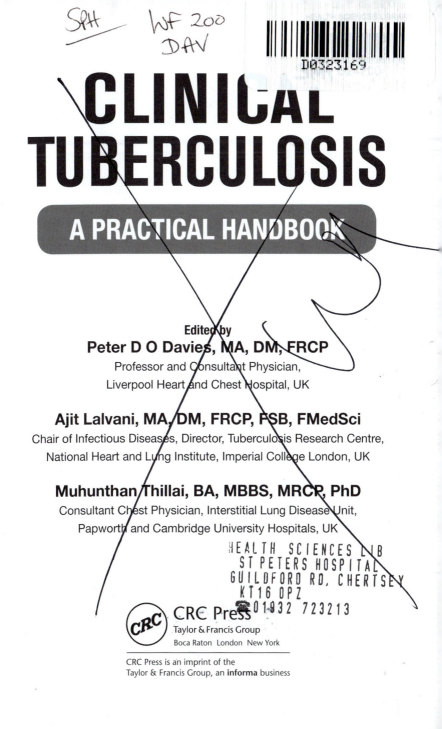

CRC Press
Taylor & Francis Group
Boca Raton London New York

CRC Press is an imprint of the
Taylor & Francis Group, an **informa** business

CRC Press
Taylor & Francis Group
6000 Broken Sound Parkway NW, Suite 300
Boca Raton, FL 33487-2742

Printed on acid-free paper
Version Date: 20151102

International Standard Book Number-13: 978-1-4441-6320-9 (Paperback)

Visit the Taylor & Francis Web site at
http://www.taylorandfrancis.com

and the CRC Press Web site at
http://www.crcpress.com

Contents

Preface

When The Global Fund, as part of its millennium goals, announced its commitment to the eradication of HIV/AIDS, tuberculosis and malaria in 2000, those of us working on tuberculosis looked forward to a time of world commitment to the eradication of the disease. We little expected that the central disease in the trio would be relatively overlooked to the benefit of the neighbours. It seems that the mass media of the world are unable to hold three things in collective memory.

There is still remarkable ignorance of tuberculosis in every part of the world, perhaps because of the stigma it still raises. I never cease to be amazed by the mistakes people of my own country make around tuberculosis, in terms of missed diagnosis, incorrect treatment and errors of disease control. In microbiology and public health, there are good standards for quality control and accepted procedures. It is the area of clinical medicine that gives me most concern. There is a belief that tuberculosis is for a small group of experts, but any and every clinician, from the paediatric abdominal surgeon to the district nurse, may meet tuberculosis in virtually any presentation. No patient group of any age, or body part, is necessarily spared from this dangerous, disabling and deadly disease. We still need to educate our doctors, nurses and other health care workers as much as we need to raise awareness among the public.

In contrast to the early 1990s when the first edition of *Clinical Tuberculosis* was published, there now seems to be no shortage of big textbooks on tuberculosis. What is lacking is a small pocket-sized book which can assist the bedside clinician to diagnose and manage cases of tuberculosis. There is a need for a book which can be carried around and referred to at any time to provide practical guidance on most aspects of the disease.

The challenge in creating this type of handbook is determining who indeed is the target reader? Should it be for the developed world where every modern test and diagnostic aid is available or for the poorest parts of the world where diagnosis can only be made by smear microscopy? Should we aim for areas of the world where tuberculosis is a rare but fascinating disease or where it is as common as the dust beneath the feet?

In this pocket book, we have tried to straddle both worlds. More is being done to help diagnosis in the poorest settings; for example diagnostic tests such as Gene-expert are now being introduced in some of the poorest parts of the world. However, that does not mean that health professionals in developed countries could not benefit from such a concise and portable reference. It is hoped that the pocket book will be of help to *all* managing tuberculosis in both the richest and poorest settings.

This book has been in evolution a long time, and I am grateful to all the authors for their patience and preparedness to write and rewrite as required. I would like to thank Dr. Jayant Banavalaker from New Delhi, Dr. Lovett Lawsen from Abuja and Dr. WW Yew from Hong Kong for their advice at an early stage in the book's development. I thank Taylor & Francis Group for taking on the publication from Hodder Arnold. I also thank the regional editors for their input. Most of all, I thank Dr. Muhunthan Thillai and Professor Ajit Lalvani for taking over the editorship in the final months, enabling me to step down towards retirement.

I hope the book proves a success not just because it will be of help to the health professional managing tuberculosis but because it will provide a means for saving lives and eventually eliminating this dreadful disease.

Peter DO Davies
Liverpool, England

Editors

Professor Peter DO Davies qualified at Oxford and St Thomas's Hospital in 1973. He was appointed as a consultant respiratory physician to Aintree Hospital and the Liverpool Heart and Chest Hospital in 1988. He is author of more than 120 peer-reviewed papers, more than 50 book chapters and 200 abstracts and 150 other articles. Professor Davies is editor of *Clinical Tuberculosis*, now in its fifth edition. In 2004, he was appointed honorary professor at Liverpool University. He is secretary of the UK-based charity TB Alert and one of two editors-in-chief of the tuberculosis section of the *International Journal of Tuberculosis and Lung Disease*.

Professor Ajit Lalvani graduated in medicine from the Universities of Oxford and London followed by further specialty training in London, Cambridge, Basel and Oxford. After his doctoral thesis, 'Immunity to Intracellular Pathogens', as a Medical Research Council (MRC) clinical research fellow at the Weatherall Institute of Molecular Medicine, he developed his research programme into tuberculosis. In 2007, he was recruited to Imperial College London to formulate new scientific and public health strategies to tackle the problem of tuberculosis worldwide. Professor Lalvani has published more than 130 peer-reviewed papers with more than 8000 citations. He has been awarded more than £15 million research funding from the Wellcome Trust, MRC, National Institute for Health Research (NIHR) and the British Lung Foundation. He is currently chair of infectious diseases at the NIHR, senior investigator at Imperial College London and honorary consultant physician at Imperial College Healthcare NHS Trust, London, United Kingdom.

Dr Muhunthan Thillai graduated from St Mary's Medical School in London in 2002. He also holds a BA in medical journalism. He undertook postgraduate training in London and Oxford before being awarded a Wellcome Trust research training fellowship, which led to a PhD in immunology and proteomics at Imperial College London, London, United Kingdom. Dr. Thillai has authored a number of scientific papers and book chapters and has edited several books. In 2014, he was appointed as consultant chest physician to the Interstitial Lung Disease Unit based in Papworth and Cambridge University Hospitals.

Contributors

Andrea M Collins
Respiratory Infection Group
Liverpool School of Tropical Medicine
and
Royal Liverpool and Broadgreen University Hospital Trust
Liverpool, United Kingdom

Manish Gautam
Department of Respiratory Medicine
Royal Liverpool University Hospital
Liverpool, United Kingdom

David KK Ho
Department of Molecular and Cellular Immunology
Institute of Child Health
University College London
London, United Kingdom

and

Department of Women's and Children's Health
University of Liverpool Institute of Translational Medicine
Alder Hey Children's NHS Foundation Trust
Liverpool, United Kingdom

Gareth H Jones
Department of Respiratory Medicine
Royal Liverpool and Broadgreen University Hospitals
Liverpool, United Kingdom

Syed Murtaza H Kazmi
Department of Respiratory Medicine
Mid-Cheshire Hospital Foundation Trust
Crewe, United Kingdom

William J Kent
Department of Respiratory Medicine
Royal Liverpool and Broadgreen University Hospitals
Liverpool, United Kingdom

Daniel Komrower
Respiratory Department
Aintree University Hospital
Liverpool, United Kingdom

Diana Lees
Department of Respiratory Medicine
Mid-Cheshire NHS Foundation Trust
Crewe, United Kingdom

Dilip Nazareth
Department of Respiratory Medicine
University Hospitals Bristol NHS Trust
and
Faculty of Health Sciences
University of Bristol
Bristol, United Kingdom

Maria Elpida Phitidis
Department of Respiratory Medicine
Wirral University Teaching Hospital NHS Foundation Trust
Wirral, United Kingdom

Rahuldeb Sarkar
Department of Respiratory Medicine and Critical Care
Medway Maritime Hospital Gillingham
Kent, United Kingdom

Gurinder Tack
Aintree Chest Centre
Aintree University Hospital
Liverpool, United Kingdom

Muhunthan Thillai
Interstitial Lung Disease Unit
Papworth and Cambridge University Hospitals
Cambridge, United Kingdom

Laura Watkins
Aintree Chest Centre
Aintree University Hospital
Liverpool, United Kingdom

1

Epidemiology

DIANA LEES

MYCOBACTERIUM TUBERCULOSIS

ORGANISMS

Tuberculosis (TB) is a communicable disease caused by a group of genetically related mycobacteria. They belong to the family Mycobacteriaceae and the order Actinomycetales and are collectively known as the *Mycobacterium tuberculosis complex*. In humans these include the following:

1. *M. tuberculosis*: The most common causative agent of human mycobacterial infection.
2. *Mycobacteruium bovis*: Historically an important causative agent of infection transmitted by unpasteurised milk, and currently found in a small percentage in developing countries.
3. *Mycobacterium africanum*: Isolated in small groups in West and Central Africa.

> **BOX 1.1: Ten important questions about current tuberculosis epidemiology**
>
> 1. What is the burden of tuberculosis (TB) worldwide and which countries are the most affected?
> 2. Why does *M. tuberculosis* cause epidemics of a rare disease over centuries?
> 3. Why do some people get TB and others do not?
> 4. Why did TB decline in Europe and North America for most of the twentieth century?
> 5. What explains the resurgence of TB since 1990, especially in Africa and former Soviet countries?
> 6. Does variation between *M. tuberculosis* strains modify the natural history, epidemiology and control of TB epidemics?
> 7. How does TB affect the distribution of other diseases?
> 8. How can current strategies be enhanced to improve the control of TB epidemics?
> 9. Will TB become resistant to all antibiotics?
> 10. How can novel tools and pharmacological interventions (such as diagnostics, drugs and vaccines) contribute to the control of TB epidemics?

4. Others include *Mycobacterium carnettii* and *Mycobacterium microti* which are also part of the complex but rarely cause infection in humans (Box 1.1).

SPREAD OF DISEASE

Mycobacteria are slow-growing acid-fast bacilli (due to the high lipid content of their cell wall). They are rod shaped, slender and slightly curved measuring $4 \times 0.3\ \mu m$. The disease is spread as a result of airborne droplet nuclei dispersed by infected individuals with active TB from their airways through coughing, singing or other activities, and these small particulates can remain suspended in the air for hours.

1. Of those exposed to an infectious individual for a considerable period, e.g. within the same household, 20%–30% will become infected.

2. Most of these primary infections resolve spontaneously but 5% will go on to develop active disease by 2 years post-exposure and a further 5% will develop the disease later on in life.

3. These figures are, however, subject to various factors that modulate the interaction between the pathogen and the host, e.g. for individuals with HIV, this risk is as high as 10% per year.

4. In active pulmonary disease, cough, sputum and haemoptysis may be a feature with other constitutional symptoms such as weight loss, fatigue, night sweats and fever.

5. Extra-pulmonary TB will produce similar constitutional symptoms as well as specific symptoms related to the site of infection.

6. Untreated sputum smear-positive cases of pulmonary TB, in the absence of HIV, results in a 70% death rate in 10 years. In smear-negative cases, 20% die within 10 years.

7. Effective treatment greatly reduces the infective risk. Strategies towards ensuring case detection and the provision of appropriate treatment are, therefore, paramount towards an effective programme aimed at reducing incidence, prevalence and death rates from the organism.

NONTUBERCULOUS MYCOBACTERIUM

ORGANISMS

Nontuberculous mycobacterium (NTM) are a group of mycobacteria which occur naturally, living in water and soil. These include *Mycobacterium kansasii, M. malmoense, M. xenophi, M. simiae* and *M. avium intracellulare*. They are not directly communicable and the disease is thought to be acquired from environmental exposure in susceptible individuals who have immunodeficiency or an underlying pulmonary disease with pre-existing cavitation.

CLINICAL PICTURE

Clinically, it most commonly presents as pneumonia but can also affect the skin, soft tissues or lymphatic drainage system. Diagnosis is based upon clinical history, radiographic findings of nodules or opacities on a plain chest radiograph and the presence of multifocal bronchiectasis, with multiple small nodules on CT (computerised tomography) scan.

MICROBIOLOGY

Microbiological confirmation is also required with two positive sputum samples, culture from bronchial wash or lavage or a transbronchial biopsy with features of granulomatous inflammation and confirmation of acid-fast bacilli. Further discussion with regard to the diagnosis and treatment of NTM is beyond the scope of this book.

HISTORICAL EPIDEMIOLOGY

HISTORICAL EVIDENCE

1. Evidence of the existence of TB has been suggested in Europe from skeletal tissue remains identified from the Neolithic period (8000–5000 BC) and also in Egyptian mummies from 1000 BC.
2. Evidence of skeletal TB has also been found in the Middle East (3000 BC), Asia and the Pacific islands (2200 BC) and North America (AD 900).
3. As populations grew and became urbanised, the incidence of TB also grew. With the advent of the Industrial Revolution by 1750, as much as 25% of all deaths in northern Europe at that time point were attributed

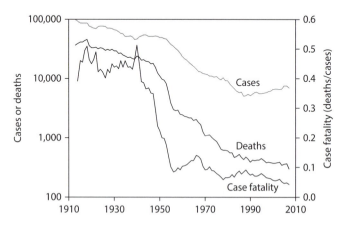

Figure 1.1 Decline in TB cases and deaths in England and Wales from 1912. Case fatality remained at 40%–50% until TB drugs became available during the 1940s; it fell sharply into the 1950s and more slowly thereafter. (Courtesy of UK Health Protection Agency.)

to TB. The disease was further spread by Europeans colonising America, South America and Africa.

4. As living conditions improved together with an increased understanding of how the disease was spread, rates slowly started to decline. Initially, infected individuals were encouraged to move to mountain or seaside climates, such that by 1850, sanatoria were encouraged.

5. This isolation of cases appears to have had an influence on the spread of the disease, but it was not until the 1940s when chemotherapy agents became widely available that the incidence began to decline. Subsequently, newer anti-TB drugs were discovered such that the rates steadily declined until the mid-1980s. Epidemiological studies suggested that the emergence of human immunodeficiency virus (HIV), immigration from areas of high prevalence, poverty and ineffective treatment programme subsequently led to resurgence of the disease with the emergence of drug resistance in some cases (Figures 1.1 and 1.2).

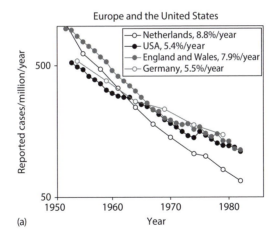

Figure 1.2 Examples of the decline in TB incidence, prevalence and mortality nationally and sub-nationally, under the influence of large-scale programmes of drug treatment. (a) Case notifications from three European countries plus the United States. (From Dye C et al., *Annu Rev Public Health*, WHO, 1980; Styblo K., *Epidemiology of Tuberculosis*, 2nd edn., KNCV Tuberculosis Foundation, The Hague, the Netherlands, 1991, p. 136; Centers for Disease Control and Prevention, Tuberculosis (TB), 2012. Available from: http://www.cdc.gov; Health Protection Agency, Tuberculosis (TB), 2012. Available from: http://www.hpa.org.uk; Styblo K et al., Tuberculosis Surveillance Research Unit, Progress Report 1, pp. 17–78, 1997.) *(Continued)*

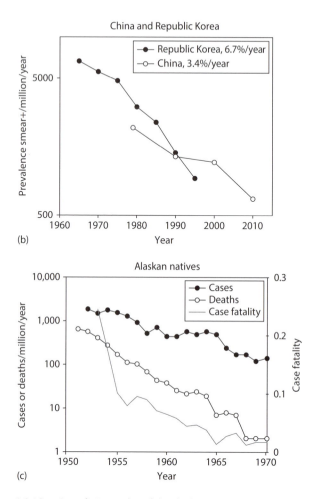

Figure 1.2 (*Continued*) Examples of the decline in TB incidence, prevalence and mortality nationally and sub-nationally, under the influence of large-scale programmes of drug treatment. (b) National population-based prevalence surveys in the Republic of Korea (1965–1995) and China (1979–2010). (From Hong YP et al., *Int J Tuberc Lung Dis*, 2, 27, 1998; China Tuberculosis Control Collaboration, *Lancet*, 364, 417, 2004; Wang L et al., Prevalence and trends in smear-positive and bacteriologically-confirmed pulmonary tuberculosis in China in 2010, unpublished, 2012.) (c) TB cases and deaths recorded from an intensively studied population of Alaskan natives (1952–1970). Case fatality is estimated as the ratio of deaths per cases. (From Grzybowski S et al., *Tubercle*, 57(Suppl.), S1, 1976.)   (*Continued*)

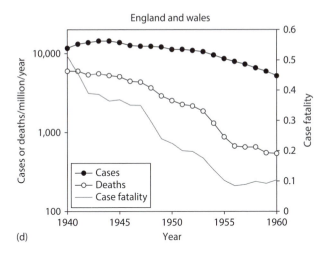

Figure 1.2 (*Continued*) Examples of the decline in TB incidence, prevalence and mortality nationally and sub-nationally, under the influence of large-scale programmes of drug treatment. (d) National case and death notifications from England and Wales, 1940–1960, with case fatality estimated as in (c). (From Health Protection Agency, Tuberculosis (TB), 2012. Available from: http://www.hpa.org.uk.)

6. It is now well established that to treat TB more than one antibiotic agent is required. Traditionally, this has been a quadruple cocktail of rifampicin, isoniazid, ethambutol and pyrazinamide.

7. The mid-1990s revealed the emergence of multidrug-resistant (MDR)-TB and extensively drug-resistant (XDR)-TB, both of which have become an important factor complicating disease prevention and control. MDR-TB is defined as TB with resistance to both rifampicin and isoniazid (the two first-line drugs) with or without resistance to other drugs. XDR-TB is MDR-TB with additional resistance to at least one fluoroquinalone and one of the second-line injectable agents of amikacin, kanamycin or capreomycin.

8. Individuals at highest risk of developing MDR-TB and XDR-TB are those who previously received treatment for TB but were non-compliant or did not complete their treatment. Those who have previously been treated for TB are at a five times higher risk of developing resistant strains than those who are newly diagnosed. Travel to or emigration from areas of higher incidence of MDR-/XDR-TB also increases an

individual's risk of infection. Co-infection with HIV and poverty may also increase the risk.

9. Historical epidemiological data have helped to improve our understanding of disease patterns, resistance profiles and reasons for its spread and has allowed us to tailor approaches towards the control of the burden of disease.

CURRENT GLOBAL BURDEN OF DISEASE

The World Health Organisation (WHO) collects data annually with regard to the incidence and prevalence of TB globally, including the number of new cases, age, sex and the rates of concomitant HIV infection.

REPORTING

1. Reporting is voluntary and as such the quality of the data can vary. To overcome this, two sets of figures are reported, that is the actual number of reported cases by each country together with an estimated number of cases. It is the estimated figure that takes precedence.

2. Epidemiology of the disease varies around the world and individual data for each country is currently available on the WHO website at http://www.who.int/tb/country/en/.

3. According to the 16th WHO global report, it is estimated that one-third of the world's population, or two billion people, are currently infected with TB. In 2010, there were 8.8 million new cases and 1.4 million deaths, including 350,000 deaths in patients co-infected with HIV.

4. Men were more likely than women to have the disease and two-thirds of notified cases were those aged 15–59 years.

FIGURES BY COUNTRY

1. Ninety-six countries currently account for 89% of the world's TB cases with the highest rates of TB in sub-Saharan Africa, India, China and Southeast Asia. In sub-Saharan Africa, the rate is as high as 276/100,000 new cases per year. In the 1990s, sub-Saharan Africa and the former Soviet Union demonstrated the largest rises in TB incidence, despite falling numbers elsewhere in the world (Figures 1.3 and 1.4).

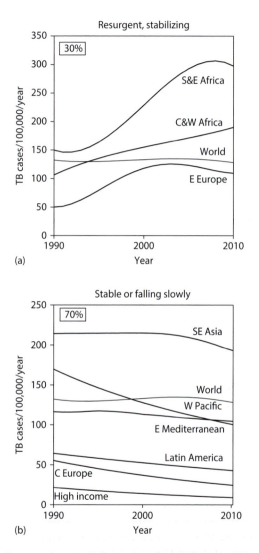

(a)

(b)

Figure 1.3 Estimated case incidence rates for (a) three regions in which TB has been resurgent, but incidence has begun to stabilise, and (b) six regions in which incidence has been stable or falling slowly. For comparison, thin lines in each panel show the trend for the whole world. (Derived from World Health Organization, Global tuberculosis control: WHO report 2011, WHO, Geneva, Switzerland, 2011.)

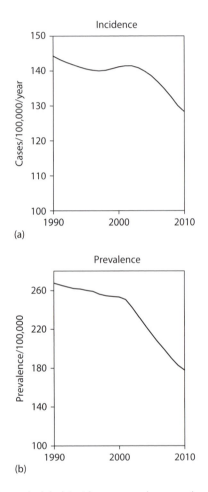

Figure 1.4 Estimated global incidence, prevalence and mortality rates for all forms of TB per 100,000 population, 1990–2010. Mortality and incidence rates are per year. Note the different scales on the vertical axes. (a) Incidence, (b) prevalence. (Derived from World Health Organization, Global tuberculosis control: WHO report 2011, WHO, Geneva, Switzerland, 2011.)   (*Continued*)

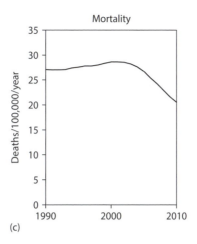

(c)

Figure 1.4 (Continued) Estimated global incidence, prevalence and mortality rates for all forms of TB per 100,000 population, 1990–2010. Mortality and incidence rates are per year. Note the different scales on the vertical axes. (c) mortality. (Derived from World Health Organization, Global tuberculosis control: WHO report 2011, WHO, Geneva, Switzerland, 2011.)

2. In 2010, there were approximately 1.4 million deaths worldwide from TB, almost a quarter of which were in patients with HIV co-infection. After HIV/AIDS, TB is the greatest global killer among infectious diseases.

3. In 2010, 59% of estimated cases were in Asia and 26% in Africa. In total, 22 countries that have been deemed to be high burden countries account for 81% of all estimated cases worldwide. Among these countries, five have the largest number of incidence and are as follows:
   a. India: 2–2.5 million
   b. China: 0.9–1.2 million
   c. South Africa: 0.4–0.59 million
   d. Indonesia: 0.37–0.54 million
   e. Pakistan: 0.33–0.48 million

4. Combined, India and China account for 38% of all TB cases worldwide, and India accounts for 26%. The lowest rates are found in Western Europe, Canada, United States and Australia where there are <25/100,000 new cases per year.

5. In 2009, out of the 250,000 cases reported of MDR-TB, 58 were in the United Kingdom, and between 2005 and 2008, 5 cases of XDR-TB were reported. In 2008, there were an estimated 440,000 cases of MDR-TB globally with 150,000 deaths. The WHO estimates that 5.4% of MDR-TB cases would in fact be XDR-TB.

CONTROL STRATEGIES

1. Following the World Health Assembly in 1991, TB was recognised as a major health problem and in 1993 the WHO declared TB to be a 'Global Emergency'.
2. In response to this, the WHO developed the Directly Observed Therapy Strategy (DOTS) in the mid-1990s. This was subsequently followed by its Stop TB Partnership with the aim of eliminating TB through improving diagnostics and treatments to produce a more effective vaccine than BCG and the expansion of the DOTS alone.
3. Since 2002 TB incidence rates have been falling and the absolute number of new cases has been decreasing since 2006 but the overall decline per capita has been slow (1%–2% per year).
4. It is now well established that poverty, HIV and the emergence of drug resistance have contributed to the resurgence of TB globally and as such efforts have been made to include these factors into strategies towards diagnosing, treating and controlling its spread. The clear aims set out by the Millennium Development Goals (MDG) are, however, unlikely to be met:
   a. Halt and reverse the rising incidence of TB by 2015
   b. Halve the prevalence of TB and death rates by 2015
   c. Ultimately reduce the global incidence rate of active disease to <1 per 1 million population per year, which would effectively eliminate TB as a public health problem.
5. Beyond 2015, the aim is to eliminate TB by the year 2050 (i.e. <1 new case per million population), but currently with the available control strategies, this target too seems ambitious.
6. It has been predicted that it would be necessary to detect at least 70% of incident cases of infectious TB and to cure at least 85% of those cases in order to reduce the incidence, prevalence and deaths attributable to TB in order to reach these goals.

7. The DOTS strategy has five major components:
    a. To secure political commitment towards financing the development of national and international partnerships with increased and sustained financing in order to develop long-term plans for TB control programmes.
    b. Improve case detection in symptomatic patients through quality assured bacteriology by providing a wide network of well-equipped laboratories using national standards for identifying the disease in accordance with international guidelines.
    c. To provide standardised treatment and, where necessary, provide supervised treatment. Treatment choices should be made in accordance with WHO guidance of treatment choice and length to reduce the risk of drug resistance.
    d. To ensure an uninterrupted and sustained supply of quality-assured anti-TB drugs, free to all TB patients.
    e. To develop an effective monitoring and evaluation system so that data can be compiled and analysed with regard to patient data and treatment outcomes. The epidemiological data can then be scrutinised with regard to the burden and the impact interventions to control TB have upon incidence, prevalence and mortality.
8. Between 1995 and 2010, 55 million people have been treated under the DOTS programme and of these 46 million were successfully treated. Data from 2009 revealed a treatment success rate of 87%.
9. Following the implementation of this strategy, challenges that had not been fully appreciated emerged and subsequent strategies have been developed to further the advancement of the WHO aims for 2015 and 2050. For instance, in countries with a high rate of HIV, most notably in Sub-Saharan Africa, the targets set out by the Stop TB strategy are unlikely to be met. Consequently, one of the components set out by the Stop TB strategy now includes increased collaboration between TB and HIV control activities. Other areas included in the updated strategy are as follows:
    a. Expansion and enhancement of the DOTS strategy
    b. Strategies to mange MDR-TB
    c. Address the needs of TB contacts and those of the poor and vulnerable
    d. Improve health-care strategies, with regard to primary care

e. Engaging health-care providers through community programmes and towards developing international standards for care
f. Empower those with TB through improved communication, social mobilisation, improving health promotion and prevention of disease
g. Encourage research with a view to developing new drugs, diagnostics and vaccines

10. The WHO has issued guidance for each of these new strategies and can be found on the website http://www.who.int/tb/strategy/en/. These strategies are designed to encourage the implementation of international standards for treatment. Where rates of MDR/XDR-TB are high, drug susceptibility testing is recommended to ensure that individuals are given appropriate therapy with the highest chance of cure. It is, therefore, necessary to ensure that laboratories are appropriately equipped to deal with testing and rapid diagnostics.

SUMMARY

1. One-third of the world's population is estimated to be infected with TB. Incidence rates have been falling since 2002 and the absolute number of new cases has been decreasing since 2006.
2. TB is the eighth leading cause of death worldwide (1.4 million in 2010) and the second leading cause of death due to an infectious agent behind HIV.
3. Ninety-six countries currently account for 89% of the world's TB cases. Twenty-two countries have been deemed to be high burden countries as they account for 81% of all estimated cases worldwide.
4. The WHO and Millennium Development Goals have set targets to halt and reverse the rising incidence of TB by 2015, halve the prevalence of TB and death rates by 2015 and ultimately to reduce the global incidence rate of active disease to <1 per 1 million population per year, which would effectively eliminate TB as a public health problem.
5. The DOTS strategy was developed in the mid-1990s in response to the global resurgence of TB and have subsequently been built upon to improve working partnerships towards reaching those targets in the MDG and to encompass strategies against new threats towards TB control and treatment programmes.
6. HIV, poverty, limited access to quality health care and MDR/XDR-TB are the biggest threats to achieving the aims of the MDG.

FURTHER READING

BMRC. Streptomycin treatment of pulmonary tuberculosis. *BMJ* 1948;2:769–782.

Davies P, Barnes P, Gordon SB. *Clinical Tuberculosis.* CRC Press, Boca Raton, FL, 2008, pp. 3–41.

Diagnosis and treatment of disease caused by nontuberculous mycobacteria: The official statement of the American thoracic society. *Am J Crit Care Med* 1997;152:S1–S25.

Dye C et al. Prospects for worldwide tuberculosis control under the WHO DOTS strategy. Directly observed short course therapy. *Lancet* 1998;352:1886.

Fauci AS et al. *Harrisons Principles of Internal Medicine*, CRC Press, Boca Raton, FL, Vol. 1. 1998, pp. 1004–1019.

WHO Global TB report. http://who.int/tb/dots/en/. Accessed 2012.

WHO Global TB report. http://www.who.int/tb/country/en/. Accessed 2012.

Jasmer RM et al. Latent tuberculoses infection. *N Engl J Med* 2002; 347:1860–1866.

Lopez AD et al. *Global Burden of Disease and Risk Factors.* Oxford University Press/The World Bank, New York, 2006.

Nelson KE, Williams CM. *Infectious Disease Epidemiology Theory and Practice*, CRC Press, Boca Raton, FL, 2nd edn. 2007.

Raviglione MC, Uplekar M. WHO's new stop TB strategy. *Lancet* 2006;367:952–955.

Stop TB Partnership. The global plan to stop TB 2011–2015. Transforming the fight towards elimination of TB, 2010.

World Health Organisation. Forty-fourth world health assembly. WHO, Geneva, Switzerland, 1991.

World Health Organisation. Multi drug and extensively multi-drug resistant TB (M/XDR-TB): 2010 global report on surveillance and response. WHO/HTM/TB/2010.3. WHO, Geneva, Switzerland, 2009.

World Health Organisation. WHO global tuberculosis control report 2010. WHO/HTM/TB/2010.07. WHO, Geneva, Switzerland, 2010.

World Health Organisation Global Tuberculosis Control. 2011.

Zignol M et al. Global incidence of multi-drug resistant tuberculosis. *J Infect Dis* 2006;194:479.

2

Pathophysiology, microbiology and immunopathology

WILLIAM J KENT

PATHOPHYSIOLOGY

CLASSICAL TUBERCULOID GRANULOMA

1. The initial response to infection with *Mycobacterium tuberculosis* (MTB) is the formation of a granuloma.
   a. A granuloma is an organised collection of activated macrophages.
   b. Macrophages differentiate from monocytes and are the most effective phagocytic cells in the body.
   c. A macrophage is 'activated' by cytokines (predominantly interferon-γ [IFN-γ]) in response to the antigen (in this case, antigen triggers from MTB).
   d. The macrophage then undergoes morphological changes, such as development of a large pale-staining round or elongated nucleus. These cells are sometimes termed epithelioid cells due to their resemblance to epithelial cells.

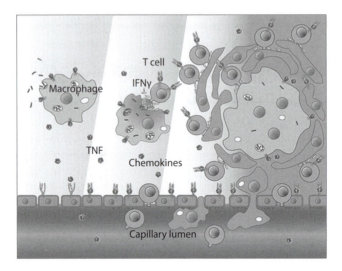

Figure 2.1 Granuloma formation in the lung. The central region of multinu-cleated giant cells, mycobacteria and necrotic debris (right) is surrounded by concentric rings of tightly apposed epithelioid cells and lymphocytes, with smaller numbers of neutrophils, plasma cells and fibroblasts.

    e. Granulomas may also contain multinucleated giant cells, such as the Langerhans giant cell. Similar to activated macrophages, these cells have increased enzymatic activity and also function as antigen presenting cells.

    f. Langerhans cells are often associated with MTB; however, they can occur in most granulomatous diseases (Figures 2.1 and 2.2).

2. Macrophages are not the only cells to be associated with granulomas, and can include lymphocytes, neutrophils, fibroblasts and eosinophils amongst others. This is often variable depending on the underlying nature of the disease.

3. In tuberculosis, granulomas aggregate to form larger masses and classically undergo necrosis to give a yellow appearance. It is this characteristic that results in the term 'caseous' (cheese-like) granuloma.

NATURAL HISTORY OF MTB INFECTION

1. The course of MTB infection and disease has several distinct stages and can lead to a variety of clinical presentations.

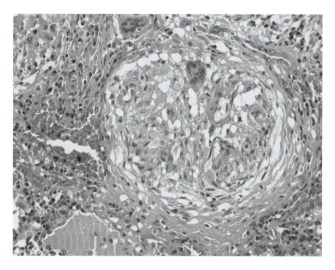

Figure 2.2 Microscopic appearance of a well circumscribed, non-caseating granuloma composed of epithelioid cells with a single giant cell. Fibrosis is seen at the periphery of the granuloma in the lower half of the picture.

2. The majority of immunocompetent MTB-infected individuals do not go on to develop TB disease in their lifetime.
3. It is likely that immune mechanisms, as yet not fully characterised, suppress latent foci of infection that do not become clinically apparent unless the immune system is compromised.

INITIAL INFECTION

1. Infection usually occurs as a result of inhalation of an infective aerosol of droplet nuclei that contain MTB, transmitted from an infected individual.
2. Transmitted organisms are then deposited within the terminal bronchioles of the exposed patient. At this stage, the infection may be cleared or latent TB infection may be induced, and the frequency with which this happens is not known.
3. The risk of developing latent infection from a smear-positive contact increases with the length and intensity of exposure.
4. Household contacts usually have a 30%–50% chance of acquiring TB infection as evidenced by a positive tuberculin skin test (TST), MTB

antigen-specific lymphocyte proliferation or interferon gamma release assay (IGRA).

5. The risk is increased in confined environments such as overcrowded housing or prisons.
6. Of the exposed patients that develop latent TB, 5%–10% develop active TB during their lifetime.
7. Those that are infected in infancy, adolescence or old age are more likely to progress to active infection.
8. It is also possible to develop TB infection following deposition within the oropharynx or intestine, or via inoculation to the skin. Tuberculosis verrucosa cutis, also known as 'prosector's wart', is associated with professions such as pathologists, butchers, anatomists and laboratory workers who handle TB-infected specimens.

Primary TB

Following arrival in the alveoli, the initial infection most often develops in subpleural locations.

1. It is assumed that an early neutrophil reaction is unable to control the spread of bacilli and that macrophages are recruited at this stage, which enable transportation to the local lymph nodes.
2. It is at this stage that macrophage aggregation occurs in lymph nodes and at the initial site of infection.
3. Caseation necrosis occurs after a few weeks, as well as the start of the T-cell response.
4. The necrosis is thought to be a combination of apoptosis of macrophages and T cells, as well as infarction via microvascular thrombosis.
5. Following exposure to MTB, most immunocompetent individuals develop an effective immune response that contains the MTB infection. The lung lesion usually heals, as do the hilar nodes and smaller peripheral foci.
6. The effect of the inflammatory response on the lung parenchyma results in a small area of fibrotic scarring that may be visible on a chest radiograph (known as a Ghon focus), and calcification can occur within this.
7. Adaptive immunity then develops in those who are immunocompetent which provides protection against re-infection.

8. Memory T cells provide immunity that often results in a long-lasting equilibrium between host and disease.

9. In areas of high prevalence, continued exposure may maintain the adaptive immunity.

10. Seeding of MTB to distant organs happens by erosion into a vessel and dissemination to organs such as the kidney, adrenals and bone marrow.

11. Depending on the levels of bacillaemia and resultant cell-mediated immune response, different clinical pictures can develop. People who do not develop an adequate immune response may develop progressive primary TB, which is most common in the young, elderly and the immunocompromised.

12. Miliary tuberculosis occurs as a result of haematogenous spread:

    a. Granulomatous lesions in miliary TB are more necrotic, with fewer or no activated macrophages (known as 'soft tubercles').

    b. This is compared to those seen with a lower-grade bacillaemia and increased cell-mediated immune response in which the lesions seen were 'hard' tubercles with few bacilli and no caseation (Figures 2.3 and 2.4).

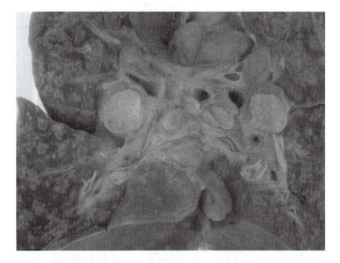

Figure 2.3 Progressive primary pulmonary tuberculosis with a view of the hilum of the lung. Multiple enlarged caseous lymph nodes are present. The lung parenchyma shows a bronchopneumonic pattern of spread with 'popcorn'-shaped lesions.

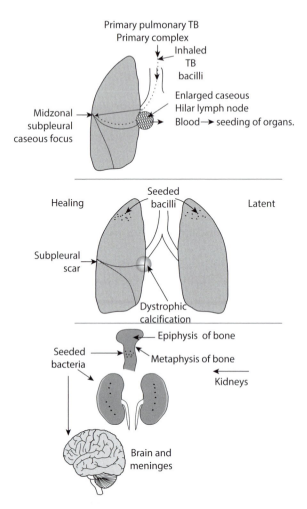

Figure 2.4 Diagram showing spread of primary tuberculosis.

Post-primary TB

Post-primary TB (PPTB) infection, i.e. tuberculous infection later in life following previous exposure, may be a result of reactivation of latent infection or re-infection.

1. The initial infection may not have been clinically apparent at the time.
2. Risk factors for further infection include the following:
   a. Increasing age
   b. Malnutrition
   c. Cirrhosis
   d. Diabetes
   e. Immunocompromise
3. Classically, tuberculous bacilli persist in the apices of the lungs due to high levels of oxygen tension. It is also thought that the lower lobes are less likely to harbour residual infection due to greater vascular supply that enables macrophages to have increased activity.
4. Bacilli also tend to be located in other areas of high oxygen tension such as the cerebral cortex, renal cortex and metaphysis of bones.
5. The source of reactivation has been investigated, and in some studies, it has been shown that healed tuberculous lesions have fewer viable bacilli than other areas of nearby macroscopically normal lung parenchyma.
6. Other studies have shown that viable bacilli are more prevalent towards the periphery of dormant lesions than in the necrotic centre.
7. PPTB classically presents as an upper zone pneumonia without hilar lymphadenopathy.
8. Compared to primary TB, the lesion usually has more parenchymal destruction and cavitation. This occurs when the lesions liquefy and the necrosis involves a bronchus.
9. Longer-term consequences of pulmonary TB can include scar-related lung cancer as a result of chronic inflammation.

MICROBIOLOGY

DIAGNOSIS

The available methods for rapid and cost-effective diagnosis of MTB remain suboptimal, particularly given the clinical challenges faced in developing countries.

1. Acid-fast smear of three expectorated sputum samples on separate days, followed by culture, remains the mainstay of diagnosis for suspected cases of pulmonary TB.
   a. However, it is estimated that only about half of all MTB cases are sputum-smear positive. This means that a significant proportion

remains undiagnosed worldwide and may present at a late stage of the disease.

b. The most appropriate initial investigation where MTB is suspected clinically is usually a chest radiograph, if available.

c. Computerised tomography (CT) scans of the chest can also provide characteristic appearances of smaller airways disease, clarify lymph node involvement and narrow the differential diagnosis.

d. Negative sputum smears do not exclude active pulmonary TB, and treatment may need to be initiated in cases of high suspicion while awaiting culture.

2. If sputum is unable to be expectorated, other options include induced sputum or fibre-optic bronchoscopy (FOB), or lymph node biopsy. Induced sputum (using hypertonic saline via a nebuliser) has been shown to be an effective way of increasing the yield of samples and has performed well in resource poor settings.

3. FOB, although semi-invasive and relatively expensive, can be extremely useful. This includes techniques such as bronchial washings, bronchoalveolar lavage, bronchial brushings and transbronchial biopsy. Samples should be sent in saline solution, as the use of preservatives such as formalin can adversely affect the sample.

4. In addition to smear and culture, FOB may provide samples for histological examination which can identify caseating granulomas and support a diagnosis of MTB. If bronchoscopy is unavailable, gastric washings may be helpful, which can identify MTB swallowed overnight.

5. Diagnosing extrapulmonary TB can be difficult and in many cases is reliant upon clinical suspicion. The principles are similar to the diagnosis of pulmonary TB, although the tests often have a lower sensitivity:

a. Lymph node biopsy of the lesion may be required, and in some cases mediastinoscopy, pleural biopsy or pus aspirated from lymph nodes can be helpful.

b. Depending on the clinical situation, CSF examination or bone marrow biopsy can also be indicated. If renal TB is suspected, early morning urine samples can be sent.

6. Tuberculin skin testing may be useful:

a. Sir Robert Koch developed an extract from sterilised MTB ('old tuberculin') that was initially thought to be a treatment for the disease. This was later found to be ineffective, but Clemens von

Pirquet, an Austrian physician, found it could be used as a skin test to detect previous TB infection.

b. Originally a drop of tuberculin was placed on the skin and a scratch made through this, but now the technique involves either intradermal injection (Mantoux test) or multiple pronged devices (Heaf test).

c. Old tuberculin has largely been replaced by alternatives such as purified protein derivative. The Mantoux test needs to be interpreted in the clinical context, e.g. ethnic origin and exposure, HIV status, immunosuppression, prior BCG vaccination. HIV co-infection may result in a false-negative TST, whereas prior BCG vaccination may result in a false-positive TST.

7. Other methods of detecting previous TB infection such as IGRAs are considered in the latent infection chapter.

Microscopy

MTB is a weak gram-positive bacilli belonging to the genus Mycobacterium.

1. MTB was first identified by Sir Robert Koch in 1882 using an alkaline-based method, which was improved upon by Paul Ehrlich who developed a more rapid technique. This involved exploiting the properties of the cell wall, which made the bacilli resistant to decolouration by acid, i.e. acid fast. This is due to high levels of mycolic acid present within them, which also makes the bacilli resistant to common antimicrobial agents (Figures 2.5 through 2.7).

2. The modification of this technique by Franz Ziehl and Friedrich Neelsen resulted in the Ziehl–Neelsen (ZN) stain, which also utilised the acid-fast properties of mycobacteria.

3. Reagents used for a ZN stain include carbol-fucshin or auramine, an acid solution (which would fail to penetrate mycobacteria), and finally a stain that allows the bacilli to be easily visualised at microscopy, such as methylene blue.

4. The ZN stain is still the most widely used stain worldwide because it is relatively inexpensive and has a long shelf life.

5. This stain has a detection threshold of approximately 5,000–10,000 bacilli/mL of sputum.

6. An alternative is the use of fluorescence microscopy, which has a slightly reduced specificity but an increased sensitivity of 10% over ZN (Figure 2.8).

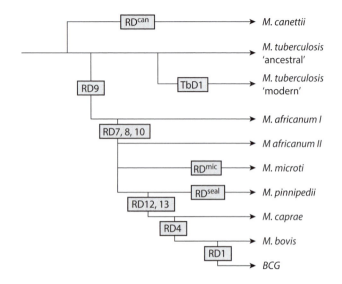

Figure 2.5 A simplified scheme of the devolutionary pathway of diversification within the *M. tuberculosis* complex. (From Davies PDO et al., *Clinical Tuberculosis*, 4th edn., CRC Press, Boca Raton, FL, 2008. With permission.)

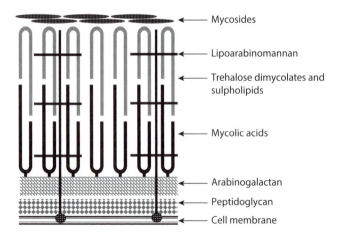

Figure 2.6 A diagrammatic representation of the mycobacterial cell wall. (From Davies PDO et al., *Clinical Tuberculosis*, 4th edn., CRC Press, Boca Raton, FL, 2008. With permission.)

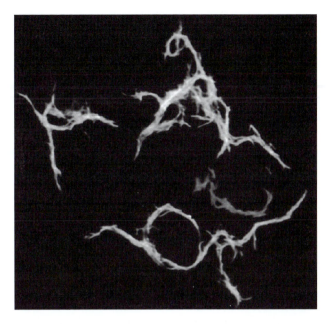

Figure 2.7 Fluorescent-stained microcolonies of *M. tuberculosis* showing cord formation. (From Davies PDO et al., *Clinical Tuberculosis*, 4th edn., CRC Press, Boca Raton, FL, 2008. With permission.)

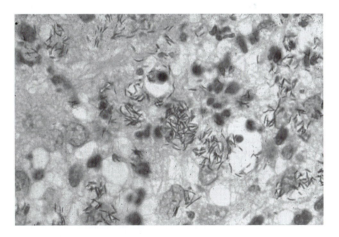

Figure 2.8 Ziehl–Neelsen stain of abundant acid-fast bacilli from a patient with multidrug-resistant tuberculosis.

CULTURE

1. *M. tuberculosis* has a long division time, and even under optimum conditions, this may take approximately 16–18 hours. Clinical specimens can take 4–6 weeks to become positive, although this may be shortened using liquid culture systems.
2. Mycobacteria can be cultured on egg-based solid media, agar-based solid media or liquid media and monitored for the visual appearance of growth.
3. Patients whose sputum smear is positive for acid-fast bacilli may be potentially infectious, but this is much less likely if TB is grown on culture alone.
4. Culture is required for definitive diagnosis; however, it is not always available worldwide. Culture is important to identify the species of mycobacteria in order that patients are not treated unnecessarily.
5. In suspected pulmonary TB, three consecutive sputum samples should be sent, or other methods such as induced sputum or bronchoscopy should be sought.

SPECIMEN PREPARATION

Due to the long division time of *M. tuberculosis*, other microorganisms may outgrow it in culture media. In order to avoid this, the specimen is decontaminated.

1. The most common method uses N-acetyl-L-cysteine–sodium hydroxide–sodium citrate. Depending on the clinical situation and the likely level of contamination, different concentrations of the reagent may be used.
2. As a higher strength of decontamination can reduce the culture rates of mycobacteria, an optimum level needs to be found in order to avoid reducing the sensitivity of culture.
3. Cross-contamination between specimens has also been shown to be a problem previously, and any suspected cases can be investigated using molecular fingerprinting methods such as restriction fragment length polymorphism (RFLP) analysis.

DIAGNOSIS OF ENVIRONMENTAL/NONTUBERCULOUS MYCOBACTERIA

1. Nontuberculous mycobacteria (NTM) are sometimes described as mycobacteria other than those of the *M. tuberculosis* complex which comprises MTB, *Mycobacterium bovis*, *Mycobacterium africanum* and

Mycobacterium microti. Other descriptions include atypical or opportunistic mycobacteria.

2. There are many different species which are found in a number of sources including soil, dust, water and milk, animals and birds. They are usually low-grade pathogens in humans, and therefore, their isolation needs to be interpreted in clinical circumstances. This includes HIV and immune status, other co-morbidities, site and frequency of culture.

3. Disease is usually only seen in patients with pre-existing lung disease or immunocompromise. The most common NTM are *Mycobacterium kansaii*, *Mycobacterium malmoense*, *Mycobacterium xenopi* and *Mycobacterium avium* complex (which includes *M. avium*, *M. intracellulare* and *M. scrofulaceum*).

4. NTM can have shorter division times than *M. tuberculosis*, and while patients are less commonly smear positive, the culture time is often shorter.

NUCLEIC ACID AMPLIFICATION TECHNIQUES

Timely diagnosis of *M. tuberculosis* is important in order to treat the disease as early as possible as well as limit the transmission of infection. Given the long periods needed for culture, techniques that provide rapid diagnosis are desirable.

1. Nucleic acid amplification tests or direct amplification tests can provide a faster diagnosis that is more sensitive and specific than smear microscopy. They are more expensive; however, they have less sensitivity and would not replace the need for traditional culture due to the need for susceptibility testing.

2. Other techniques for rapid diagnosis have shown promise in recent years including serodiagnosis and biochemical markers, PCR and phage-based assays.

3. Given the pressure on resources for all healthcare systems, in particular those in which TB is most prevalent, an ideal rapid diagnostic technique would need to be economical as well as sensitive and specific.

4. In some developing countries, standard staining and microscopy of samples (without culture) remains the only cost-effective way of rapid diagnosis.

DRUG RESISTANCE

1. Susceptibility testing is becoming ever more important due to the increasing prevalence of multidrug-resistant (MDR) TB.

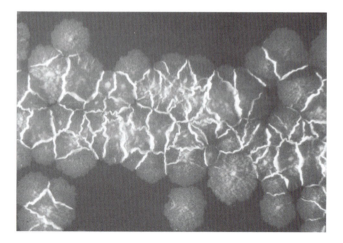

Figure 2.9 Rough colonies of *M. tuberculosis*. (Courtesy of G. Pfyffer von Altishofen, Lucerne, Switzerland.)

2. At specialised centres, there are a number of methods of rapid resistance testing such as PCR, microarray or DNA sequencing.
3. It is important to identify those at risk of MDR-TB, such as contact with a known case or those previously treated for TB, as traditional methods of susceptibility testing can take several weeks (Figure 2.9).

MTB GENOTYPING

1. The genome of MTB was first published in 1998 and the use of DNA fingerprinting can be used to subdivide MTB into different 'strains'. This has a number of clinical applications and can allow phenotypical differences to be evaluated.
2. It can be useful to separate newly acquired infections and reactivations and to link clusters of cases that other methods have failed to identify. There are several polymorphic sequences of DNA that have been described, with IS *6110* being shown to have one of the most distinctive patterns that can be compared.
3. With better clarification of related cases, those at increased risk of transmission can be identified.

4. Cross-contamination within the laboratory can also be investigated by this method, as well as helping to characterise the epidemiology and mechanisms of drug resistance.

IMMUNOPATHOLOGY

INNATE IMMUNITY

1. Following inhalation of the infective aerosol, Toll-like receptors are stimulated on monocytes, macrophages and dendritic cells, and MTB is ingested within these cells.
2. Other receptors that have been demonstrated to recognise and bind to MTB include complement receptors, the mannose receptor, CD14, surfactant protein A receptors and scavenger receptors.
3. Following the ingestion of MTB within macrophages and dendritic cells, antigens are processed and presented via the major histocompatibility complex (MHC) class I or II molecules to $CD8^+$ and $CD4^+$ T cells, respectively, as well as via other mechanisms.
4. This process initiates a signal transduction pathway that stimulates the production of cytokines and chemokines that attract other innate immune cells to the areas of infection and provides a link between the innate and adaptive immune systems.

MONOCYTES AND MACROPHAGES

1. Macrophages play a crucial role in the immune response against MTB and are mainly activated by IFN-γ.
2. Along with infected monocytes and respiratory epithelial cells, macrophages can release nitric oxide that is able to kill MTB at low concentrations.
3. Other mechanisms include acidification of the phagosome and fusion with lysosomes, although MTB may be able to avoid elimination by inhibiting these events.
4. Macrophages and monocytes undergo apoptosis (programmed cell death) in response to infection with MTB. It is thought that this is a protective mechanism to prevent the spread of mycobacteria, and it has been shown that virulent strains have been able to suppress this process.

Dendritic cells

1. Dendritic cells are potent antigen-presenting cells and are able to activate $CD4^+$ and $CD8^+$ T cells.
2. They also influence the differentiation of naïve T cells to T_H1 and T_H2 subtypes.
3. It appears that the ability of dendritic cells to inhibit growth of MTB may not be as effective as that of macrophages.

Natural killer cells

1. Natural killer (NK) cells have a variety of roles in immunity against MTB. They are able to produce T_H1 and T_H2 cytokines, IFN-γ and IL-13 and contribute to the regulation of macrophages and $CD8^+$ T cell effector function.
2. They also have bactericidal effects via direct NK-mediated killing which requires cell to cell contact.

Adaptive immunity

1. T cells play a key role in the adaptive immune response against MTB. $CD4^+$ T cells (T helper cells) release cytokines, inhibit MTB growth in monocytes and initiate and maintain the activity of $CD8^+$ cytotoxic T-cell responses.
2. The vital role of $CD4^+$ T cells is clear in HIV-1 infection as reduced $CD4^+$ T cell number and function is the greatest known risk factor for reactivation of TB or progression of primary infection to active disease.
3. When activated, $CD4^+$ T cells are able to differentiate into T_H1 and T_H2 cells.
4. Depending on the cytokines produced, a different balance of immune response can be generated. T_H1 cells secrete IFN-γ, IL-2 and TNF-α, and T_H2 cells produce IL-4, IL-5 and IL-13. In response to MTB infection, most individuals produce a predominantly T_H1 immune response.
5. $CD8^+$ cytotoxic T cells (T killer cells) predominantly act as cytotoxic T cells in the immune response, although there is some overlap in function with $CD4^+$ cells.

6. Upon interaction with an infected cell, enzymes such as granzyme and molecules such as granulysin and perforin are able to induce apoptosis. After infection with MTB, effector memory T cells are produced that can generate a rapid response to infection in peripheral sites of infection.

7. Central memory T cells need more time to regenerate an immune response and are generally maintained in lymphoid organs. These cells can expand their population in response to re-infection.

REGULATION OF T-CELL RESPONSE

1. Successful containment of MTB infection has been associated with a predominantly T_H1 response, with a key role played by IFN-γ in maintaining this balance.

2. There are several potential mechanisms by which this response can be altered, including chronic infections with parasites. This has been shown to produce a more dominant T_H2 response which can result in increased susceptibility to MTB infection.

3. Regulatory T cells (Tregs) play a vital role in the downregulation of the immune system. Their role has been shown to be important in a wide number of scenarios including autoimmune diseases, cancer and organ transplantation.

4. Tregs are able to reduce tissue damage by maintaining appropriate immune response to pathogens and auto-antigens. Tregs are a specific T-cell subset and were previously known as T suppressor cells. They have been shown to reduce T-cell proliferation and T_H1 and T_H2 responses.

5. The role of Tregs in response to MTB infection is not yet known, particularly the abilities of MTB to inhibit apoptosis of infected cells. It is not clear whether the activity of Tregs at infective sites contributes to the proliferation of MTB and ongoing infection.

MTB AND PROTECTIVE HUMAN IMMUNITY

1. In the majority of individuals, MTB infection is not fully eradicated, although it may be successfully contained by the immune response. This would suggest that MTB is able to alter the immune response, possibly at multiple levels, or remain undetected by it to promote chronic infection.

2. It has also been shown that MTB strains can differ in their virulence and in the immune response that they induce.
3. Genetic variation within a population may also be a contributing factor to the susceptibility to MTB infection.

CONDITIONS FAVOURING PROGRESSION OF MTB INFECTION

1. As mentioned previously, one of the most important co-infections that favour progression to infection is HIV-1 infection, which is covered elsewhere.
2. Inhibitors of TNF-α, such as infliximab, have been shown to increase the risk of TB reactivation. This has become increasingly important in recent years due to their widespread use in the treatment of conditions such as rheumatoid arthritis and Crohn's disease.
3. TNF-α is essential for granuloma formation and the prevention of TB reactivation. Infliximab also has effects on IFN-γ production which may increase susceptibility further.

SUMMARY

PATHOLOGY

1. The initial response to MTB infection is granuloma formation. Granulomas aggregate to form larger masses and classically undergo necrosis to give a 'caseous' (cheese-like) appearance.
2. The course of MTB infection and disease has several distinct stages and clinical presentations.
3. The majority of MTB-infected individuals do not go on to develop clinically apparent disease in their lifetime.
4. The initial infection may be cleared initially or latent TB may develop.
5. Most immunocompetent individuals develop an effective immune response that contains MTB infection. The resultant area of fibrotic scarring may be visible on a CXR (Ghon focus). Adaptive immunity develops to protect against re-infection.
6. Tuberculous infection that occurs later in life, following previous exposure, is known as post-primary infection. This may be a result of the reactivation of latent infection or re-infection.

7. Risk factors for post-primary infection include increasing age, malnutrition, cirrhosis, diabetes and immunocompromise.
8. Post-primary TB classically presents as an upper zone pneumonia without hilar lymphadenopathy.

MICROBIOLOGY

1. Acid-fast smear of three expectorated sputum samples on separate days remains the mainstay of diagnosis for suspected cases of pulmonary TB.
2. Negative sputum smears do not exclude active TB, although they are less likely to be infectious
3. A chest radiograph is usually the most appropriate initial investigation where available.
4. Computerised tomography of the chest can be helpful in the investigation of suspected cases.
5. Induced sputum, FOB or lymph node biopsy may provide samples for staining and culture.
6. Diagnosing extrapulmonary TB can be difficult and may rely on clinical suspicion. The principles of investigation are similar to pulmonary TB and the means of diagnosis can include lymph node biopsy, mediastinoscopy or pleural biopsy.
7. Staining utilises high mycolic acid content of the MTB cell wall, which makes them resistant to decolouration by acid, i.e. acid fast.
8. MTB has a long division time and culture of clinical specimens may take 4–6 weeks to become positive. Culture is important for definitive diagnosis and to exclude NTM; however, this is not universally available.
9. A number of rapid diagnostic techniques have shown promise in recent years, such as nucleic acid amplification, serodiagnosis and biochemical markers, PCR and phage-based assays.
10. Susceptibility testing can be achieved by a number of methods including PCR, microarray and DNA sequencing.

IMMUNOPATHOLOGY

1. Macrophages play a crucial role in the immune response against MTB and are mainly activated by IFN-γ. Mechanisms of action include the release of nitric oxide, acidification of phagosome and fusion with lysosomes. Macrophages undergo apoptosis in response to infection with MTB, which can prevent the spread of mycobacteria.

2. Dendritic cells also play a role in antigen presentation of MTB and influence the differentiation of naïve T cells.

3. NK cells contribute to the regulation of macrophages and T cells and also have direct bactericidal effects.

4. CD4+ (T helper cells) are able to release cytokines, inhibit MTB growth in monocytes and initiate and maintain the activity of CD8+ cytotoxic cells (T killer cells).

5. After infection with MTB, effector memory T cells produce a rapid response to infection in peripheral sites while central memory T cells expand their population.

6. The successful containment of MTB infection has been associated with a predominantly T_H1 response with IFN-γ playing a key role. Regulatory T (Treg) cells have been shown to play a vital role in the downregulation of immune system and reduction of tissue damage, and their role in MTB infection is an area of ongoing research.

7. In the majority of individuals, MTB infection is not fully eradicated, which would suggest that MTB is able to alter the immune response possibly at multiple levels or remain undetected by it to promote chronic infection.

FURTHER READING

Davies PDO, Gordon GB, Davies G. *Clinical Tuberculosis*, 5th edn. CRC Press, Boca Raton, FL, 2014.

Dheda K, Schwander SK, Zhu B, van Zyl-Smit RN, Zhang Y. The immunology of tuberculosis: From bench to bedside. *Respirology* 2010 Apr;15(3):433–450.

Hepple P1, Ford N, McNerney R. Microscopy compared to culture for the diagnosis of tuberculosis in induced sputum samples: A systematic review. *Int J Tuberc Lung Dis* 2012 May;16(5):579–588.

Gagneux S et al. Variable host-pathogen compatibility in Mycobacterium tuberculosis. *Proc Natl Acad Sci USA* 2006 Feb 21;103(8):2869–2873.

Pai M, Minion J, Steingart K, Ramsay A. New and improved tuberculosis diagnostics: Evidence, policy, practice, and impact. *Curr Opin Pulm Med* 2010 May;16(3):271–284.

Shaler CR, Horvath C, Lai R, Xing Z. Understanding delayed T-cell priming, lung recruitment, and airway luminal T-cell responses in host defense against pulmonary tuberculosis. *Clin Dev Immunol* 2012;2012:628293.

Smith T. A comparative study of bovine tubercle bacilli and of human bacilli from sputum. *J Exp Med* 1898 Jul 1;3(4–5):451–511.

van Crevel R, Kleinnijenhuis J, Oosting M, Joosten LAB, Netea MG. Innate immune recognition of *Mycobacterium tuberculosis*. *Clin Dev Immunol* 2011;2011:12pp.

Wilson ML. Rapid diagnosis of Mycobacterium tuberculosis infection and drug susceptibility testing. *Arch Pathol Lab Med* 2013 Jun; 137(6):812–819.

Wilson ML. Recent advances in the laboratory detection of *Mycobacterium tuberculosis* complex and drug resistance. *Clin Infect Dis* 2011 Jun;52(11):1350–1355.

WHO. Guidelines Approved by the Guidelines Review Committee Same-Day Diagnosis of Tuberculosis by Microscopy: WHO Policy Statement. World Health Organization, Geneva, Switzerland, 2011.

3

Pulmonary disease

DILIP NAZARETH AND ANDREA M COLLINS

PATHOGENESIS OF DISEASE

1. Pulmonary or respiratory tuberculosis (TB) is the result of an infection involving any aspect of the respiratory system, i.e. lung parenchyma, pleura, lymph nodes or large airways.
2. In a typical case, the initial area of respiratory infection results in the enlargement of adjacent lymph nodes. This combination of infection and adjacent lymph node enlargement is called the Ghon complex. A successful containment of the infection results in an area of scarring and subsequent calcification called a Ghon focus.
3. Pleural effusions occur in approximately 10% of cases and are more common in adults than in children.

4. Miliary TB represents a disseminated form of the disease and may require a computerised tomography (CT) scan as up to 50% of radiographs may show no evidence of abnormality in miliary disease.

5. In the first 3 months of treatment of pulmonary TB, there may be a paradoxical worsening of radiographic features despite an improvement in the clinical state.

6. Untreated pulmonary TB has an overall mortality rate of over 50%.

7. In a small number of patients, the disease is progressive and results in pulmonary TB. This may then result in widespread disseminated disease outside of the respiratory system (Figures 3.1 and 3.2).

The medical history of a patient with suspected pulmonary TB is vital in determining the risk of the disease as well as the severity and risk of transmission to others. However, no single question will yield an answer that is pathognomonic of the disease. Rather it is a combination of a thorough history, examination and results of investigations that will elicit the correct diagnosis.

Case study 3.1

DC is a 34-year-old Caucasian UK born male who presented to his General Practitioner (GP) with an 8-week history of cough and weight loss. On direct questioning, he admitted to night sweats ('as though I had wet the bed') and chronic fatigue. The cough was productive of sputum but no blood had been seen. He was a heavy smoker of 40 cigarettes a day. His father, who was living with him, had had TB as a child and for the past 3 months had had similar symptoms to DC. Also living at home was his 30-year-old wife and their 8-month-old son. Both were well with no symptoms of cough or weight loss. Both father and son worked behind the bar of a social club for between 20 and 30 hours a week.

His GP found nothing abnormal on examination but requested a chest x-ray which was reported as showing gross abnormalities. DC was seen at the local chest clinic the next day and admitted to hospital where he was kept in a side room. Sputum was positive on direct smear for acid-fast bacilli. A diagnosis of pulmonary TB was made and he was started on quadruple therapy. A gene probe available 2 days later showed the bacterium to be *Mycobacterium tuberculosis* with no rifampicin or isoniazid resistance. The contact tracing team visited the home and the father, wife and son attended the chest clinic. The father was found to have extensive pulmonary TB with middle

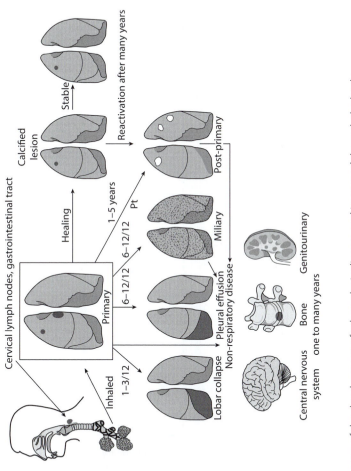

Figure 3.1 Diagram of the development of tuberculosis disease and its spread through the body.

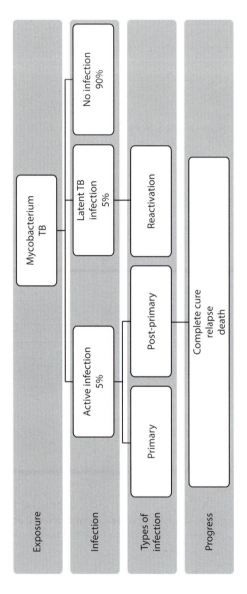

Figure 3.2 Pathogenesis of TB infection.

lobe collapse on the chest x-ray and a strongly positive Mantoux test (25 mm) on a background of no previous BCG vaccination.

At about the same time, a 50-year-old man presented to the same hospital with a large right-sided pleural effusion. He had had a few days of malaise and pleuritic chest pain but no weight loss or night sweats. The fluid was aspirated and sent for acid-fast bacilli (AFB) stain and culture. No bacteria were seen on direct microscopy but *M. tuberculosis* grew from the fluid by the 10th day of incubation. When seen by the contact investigation team, it was found that this man also worked as a barman in the social club. All 30 part-time and full-time bar staff were screened for TB by interferon-gamma release assay (IGRA) and chest radiograph. Four further cases of pulmonary TB were discovered. All four hundred members of the club were then screened. No further active cases were discovered.

HISTORY

CURRENT SYMPTOMS

1. *Cough*: This is the most common symptom in pulmonary TB and is present in over 80% of cases. It is caused by irritation of the airways due to inflammation. It is also the most common symptom of any upper or lower respiratory tract infection. The cough from pulmonary TB is often prolonged, and in any patient with a cough for more than 3 weeks, TB should be considered. In a smoker, an important differential diagnosis of a prolonged cough is lung carcinoma.
2. *Sputum production*: The cough from TB may be dry initially but if it continues sputum production may be profuse, amounting to many cupfuls in a day. In this way, TB can mimic bronchiectasis. The sputum may be clear, purulent or blood stained.
3. *Haemoptysis*: This may occur at any stage in TB but is usually associated with extensive lung destruction. In some cases, it may be profuse (over a litre) and life threatening. Haemoptysis can occur with any lung infection and pulmonary embolus and is also a common result in carcinoma.
4. *Chest pain*: This is not a common symptom of TB. It arises from the involvement of the chest wall or mediastinum where pain receptors are located rather than the lung substance itself.
5. *Breathlessness*: This may occur in advanced disease either where there is extensive lung destruction or where there is limited destruction in the

presence of some underlying alternative lung pathology such as chronic obstructive pulmonary disease.

6. *Weight loss*: This is a common systemic symptom of TB. Because the disease may be very slow in onset, the patient may lose up to a third of body mass by the time presentation occurs.

7. *Malaise*: Because of the slow onset, the patient may not realise they have become ill for some time after the onset of disease. This may present as a history of several months of malaise and fatigue.

8. *Night sweats*: They may typically be profuse and frequent. Though characteristic of TB, they may occur in many other disease causing pyrexia especially lymphoma, which is an important differential diagnosis.

PAST MEDICAL HISTORY

The past medical history should be geared towards asking questions relevant to TB with specific emphasis on associations which are recognised as risk factors for developing the disease.

1. HIV infection is the greatest risk factor in incurring TB infection and for that infection to progress to active disease. It is estimated that a HIV-negative individual infected with TB has only a 10% lifetime chance of developing disease but if co-infected with HIV has a 10% annual chance.

2. Gastrectomy or jejunostomy: A number of studies have shown that gastrectomy increases the risk of TB fivefold and jejunoileal bypass by 27–63 times. Stomach acid–reducing medication has also been shown to increase the risk of TB. The exact reasons for this are unclear.

3. Immunosuppressive and immunomodulatory drugs, e.g. TNF-alpha blockers, should be enquired about. Data on the increased risk of TB when given such immunosuppressant drugs as corticosteroids and methotrexate are anecdotal lacking hard evidence. In contrast some of the new biological compounds such as TNF-alpha blockers have been shown to increase the risk of TB by approximately eight times. Before starting such drugs, active TB and latent infection should be excluded, and most current national guidelines advise this.

4. Diabetes increases the risk of TB by between two and four times. Diabetes increases the risk of the body to most infections by non-specific reduction in immunity.

5. Carcinoma of the head and neck increases the risk of TB by 16-fold. A number of other carcinomas including lung cancer and lymphoma also increase the risk but by a lesser degree.
6. Interstitial lung diseases can increase the risk of TB by between 2- and 30-fold.

FAMILY HISTORY

1. A family history of TB is especially important when assessing the risk of TB or of diagnosing the disease. Historically, prior to isolation of mycobacteria as the cause of *Mycobacterium tuberculosis* (MTB), some societies in Europe believed that TB was a hereditary disease due to several members of the same family being diagnosed within a short period of time.
2. A number of genetic determinants have been associated with an increased risk of disease development.

SOCIAL HISTORY

1. Social factors may contribute to the development of TB and several of these are related to poverty and a low socioeconomic class.
2. Contact with smear-positive case is vital to determine as in about half of the cases of TB the patient knows someone who has the disease. In the United Kingdom, contact with a patient with active smear-positive pulmonary TB is the single most important risk factor in developing the disease. This is most often a member of the family, from whom infection has been acquired, but it is important to ask about colleagues and friends as well who may be potential sources of infection.
3. Ethnic origin is important to determine. In high-burden countries, which include most East and South Asian countries and sub-Saharan Africa, TB is still endemic, and for this reason, it is important to get a full history of both age of migration between countries and travel to countries of origin which may have higher incidence of TB.
4. Homelessness is a strong risk factor for TB in many cities and countries. In the United Kingdom, surveys in London of those sleeping on the streets have revealed a TB prevalence of up to 2%.
5. Poverty is an important risk factor for TB and a number of studies have shown a direct correlation between TB and poverty.
6. Malnutrition or a poorly balanced diet is often associated with TB.

7. Smoking is a recognised risk factor in developing TB. Studies have estimated this increased risk as two- to fivefold in smokers.
8. Alcohol consumption in excess is also a recognised risk factor in the development of TB.
9. Health-care workers are more likely to be in contact with patients with TB than members of the general public and so this may be a risk factor.

EXAMINATION

1. General appearance: Many patients with pulmonary TB will have lost weight prior to presentation so that wasting of the body tissues and musculature will be apparent.
2. Inspection of the chest, even in advanced pulmonary TB, often shows no physical abnormality.
3. Percussion of the chest may reveal dullness if there is an underlying area of consolidation or pleural effusion.
4. Auscultation may be normal over the affected area but may also reveal bronchial breathing or other signs of infection such as crepitations. A wheeze may be present over the area of endobronchial TB. This is more common in children than adults because airways are smaller and obstruction of a significant proportion of the airway diameter is more likely to occur. If there is a large cavity, amphoric breathing across the top of the cavity may be heard.
5. Signs of TB elsewhere in the body from an extra-pulmonary site may be present. It is therefore important to perform a full examination in cases of suspected pulmonary TB which should involve neurological, cardiac and abdominal examinations.

INVESTIGATIONS

BEDSIDE INVESTIGATIONS

1. Pyrexia is often present in TB, characteristically occurring in the evenings. It is usually relatively low grade, rarely rising above 39°C unless there is significant pulmonary involvement, but it is usually accompanied by profuse sweating.

2. Patients may exhibit signs of clinical infection including tachycardia and hypotension if the infection has led to sepsis.

ROUTINE BLOOD TESTS

1. There is no specific blood test that is helpful in the direct diagnosis of TB. Where resources are scarce, any blood test for TB may be unnecessary.
2. Most national guidelines from developed countries and some developing countries stipulate that a HIV test should be done on all patients diagnosed with TB.
3. Patients may have become anaemic during the course of the illness so blood tests for haemoglobin (Hb) may be needed.
4. Rarely some drugs may cause leucopoenia so that an initial white blood cell count is advisable.
5. Most guidelines require initial liver function test before treatment is started as treatment may cause hepatitic adverse events.
6. Tests for renal function are advisable, and if impaired, drug dose reduction or monitoring may be required.
7. Arterial blood gas analysis may be advisable in a patient with very advanced disease as there may be so much lung destruction that supplemental oxygen is required.

MICROBIOLOGICAL INVESTIGATIONS

1. The diagnosis of pulmonary TB infection can only be confirmed by the identification of *M. tuberculosis* complex from a specimen obtained from the patient. This is usually done by culture but polymerase chain reaction (PCR) confirmation may also be acceptable if available.
2. It is therefore imperative that good specimens of sputum are obtained for bacteriology. These are best obtained by the first morning sample of sputum.
3. Three separate samples are recommended on consecutive days if possible.
4. In the absence of adequate sputum sample, induction of sputum by inhalation of saline may be performed.
5. Alternatively, samples can be obtained by bronchoscopy and bronchial washings. This investigation may also be useful to exclude other diagnoses such as lung carcinoma.

6. If the disease appears localised to the lung parenchyma or lymph nodes, a surgical biopsy may be needed to obtain a histological diagnosis. This may require an open lung biopsy or minimally invasive techniques such as video-assisted thoracoscopic surgery.

7. Isolated airway lymph node enlargement may require histological sampling using endobronchial ultrasound techniques.

8. If the pleura is infected resulting in a pleural fluid collection, then a pleural aspirate should be performed in order to make a microbiological diagnosis. The fluid is most often an exudate. However, the sensitivity of this to make a diagnosis by identifying acid-fast bacilli is less than 10% and a pleural biopsy may be needed for histological diagnosis.

9. Samples should be collected in sterile containers and sent to the laboratory as soon as possible and clearly labelled for staining and culture for *M. tuberculosis*. Most laboratories will only carry out tests for TB if specifically asked to do so.

10. Initial staining by phenol auramine or Ziehl–Neelsen stains will show the presence of bacteria in about 50% of cases of pulmonary TB; as being relatively insensitive as a test for TB, they require over 10,000 bacteria/mL of sputum to be seen under the microscope.

11. Any mycobacterium present in enough quantities will stain to provide a positive result. Only culture or PCR will provide confirmation of the presence of *M. tuberculosis*.

12. Pulmonary infection can be caused by environmental mycobacteria such as *Mycobacterium xenopi* or *M. kansasii*, so care must be taken to positively identify the species of bacteria before the diagnosis can be confirmed. In the appropriate clinical setting, treatment may be stated whilst culture confirmation is awaited.

13. A rapid PCR test on a smear-positive sample may be available within 24–48 hours. Otherwise, liquid culture may provide an answer within 7–10 days and culture by semi-sold media in 2–6 weeks.

IMMUNE-BASED TESTS

1. IGRAs represent a relatively new type of blood test for TB. These tests are now widely available. Like the tuberculin skin test, these assays do not help differentiate latent infection from active disease. However, they may be useful in either supporting the diagnosis of active TB in patients

in whom microbiological confirmation is awaited or used as a 'rule out' test in patients at low risk of TB infection.

2. Nucleic acid amplification tests (NAATs) use techniques such as PCR to identify nucleic acid sequences in MTB within respiratory samples such as sputum by 24–48 hours. These rapid tests may be used to guide treatment whilst waiting for further culture confirmation. Advancements in testing means results are now available within a few hours.

RADIOLOGY

1. The initial test of a chest radiograph is the mainstay of investigations and in a number of instances may be the only radiographic test performed. It is also important to note that in poorly resourced settings, a chest radiograph may be an expensive and unnecessary extravagance in the scenario where a patient has sputum smear-positive disease.

2. Where chest radiography can be undertaken, it can be helpful in diagnosing smear-negative disease. There may be a characteristic pattern to post-primary pulmonary TB, though TB can present with virtually any features (Figure 3.3).

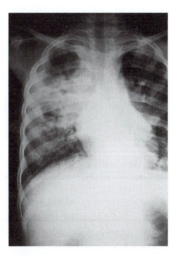

Figure 3.3 Tuberculous bronchopneumonia.

3. The most common pattern is of a soft heterogeneous shadowing predominantly in the upper lobes. Cavitation is a characteristic feature in HIV-negative disease shown as rounded areas of increased radio translucency.
4. Cavities may be of any size from a few millimetres to several centimetres. If disease is extensive, there may be destruction of the lung usually commencing with the upper lobes with progressive shadowing to all parts of the lung (Figure 3.4).
5. The radiographic features of primary TB are in contrast to those of post-primary disease. Here, there may be a small area of infection in any part of the lung, no more than a few millimetres in diameter. This is usually accompanied by proximal lymph gland enlargement presenting as hilar and/or para-tracheal gland enlargement (Figure 3.5).
6. CT may be required to further evaluate the chest looking specifically for subtle parenchymal changes, small cavities and lymph node enlargement.
7. CT may also be used in the setting of ambiguity of the diagnosis, e.g. specific features in smear-negative cases may point towards an alternative diagnosis such as sarcoidosis or lymphoma.
8. In the case of microbiologically confirmed disease, CT scans may be useful to determine the extent of disease spread, presence of cavitation and presence of co-morbid conditions such as carcinoma. CT scans may also be used in some cases as a guide to treatment response.
9. Positron emission tomography (PET) scans have been used in cases of pulmonary TB to identify lesions not seen on CT scans but their use remains unclear (Figure 3.6).

DIFFERENTIAL DIAGNOSIS OF PULMONARY TUBERCULOSIS

This is an extensive test and is related to the distribution of disease.

PARENCHYMAL DISEASE

1. Infection, e.g. bacterial, viral, and fungal
2. Carcinoma, e.g. primary lung cancer and secondary spread of cancer from other sites

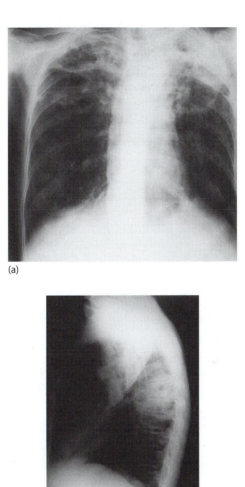

(a)

(b)

Figure 3.4 Chronic active pulmonary tuberculosis. There is extensive upper lobe fibrosis with tracheal deviation. (a) Postero-anterior view and (b) lateral view showing the posterior nature of the disease.

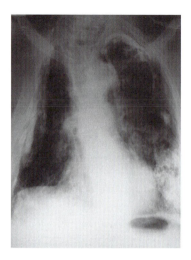

Figure 3.5 Healed (old) tuberculosis showing extensive pleural and paren-chymal calcification.

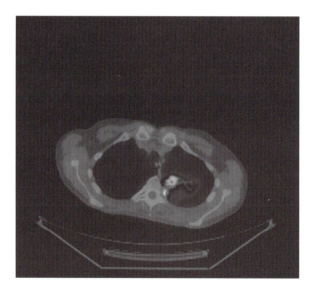

Figure 3.6 Transaxial fused PET/CT slice of upper thorax with FDG avid lesion in left upper lobe showing uptake and activity indicating ongoing infection/inflammation.

3. Sarcoidosis
4. Lymphoma
5. Interstitial lung diseases, e.g. idiopathic pulmonary fibrosis, alveolar proteinosis, and organising pneumonia

MEDIASTINAL DISEASE

1. Lymphoma
2. Cancer
3. Sarcoidosis
4. Hamartoma

PLEURAL DISEASE

1. Infection, e.g. bacterial, viral and fungal
2. Pulmonary infarction
3. Pulmonary embolus
4. Chylothorax
5. Carcinoma

MILIARY DISEASE

1. Fungal infection
2. Histoplasmosis
3. *Nocardia* infection
4. Amyloidosis
5. Post-viral infection

COMPLICATIONS OF PULMONARY TUBERCULOSIS

LOBAR COLLAPSE

1. Local lymph gland enlargement may obstruct a main bronchus causing lobar collapse.
2. If untreated, lobar collapse may result in bronchiectasis later in life.

3. The right middle lobe is commonly affected resulting in collapse. This is due to increased density of lymph nodes adjacent to this lobe in combination with the longer length of the middle lobe. This is also seen in young children and the so-called Brock's syndrome.

PLEURAL EFFUSION

1. A pleural effusion may occur 3–6 months after initial infection. It is almost always unilateral and may occupy up to two-thirds of the hemi-thorax.
2. It is usually self-limiting resolving after a few months, but in almost 50% of patients, TB of a more severe form such as post-primary pulmonary or even TB meningitis will occur within a year.
3. Diagnosis is made by pleural biopsy for culture and histology. The pleural fluid is culture positive in only a minority of cases.
4. Pleural effusions are more common in adults and more common in patients with HIV co-infection.
5. A TB empyema may occur due to an accumulation of pus in the pleural space.
6. Bronchopleural fistulae may occur due to enlarging cavities rupturing into the pleural space.

PNEUMOTHORAX

1. A pneumothorax may occur in up to 15% of patients with pulmonary TB and is more common in men and on the right side.
2. Treatment of a TB pneumothorax should follow standard treatment guidelines.

MILIARY DISEASE

This is caused by dissemination of bacteria by the blood stream or lymphatic system and is characterised by small lesions scattered throughout the whole of the lung fields as seen at radiography. Sputum is usually positive for AFB on smear but bronchoscopy, i.e. washings and biopsies for culture, and histology may be necessary to confirm the diagnosis (Figure 3.7).

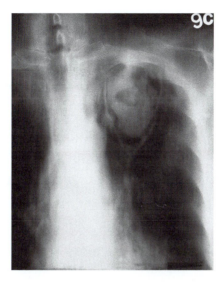

Figure 3.7 Poster anterior chest x-ray showing an aspergilloma in the left apex.

ENDOBRONCHIAL TUBERCULOSIS

This may occur due to direct infection of the bronchial wall or due to erosion from adjacent infected lymph nodes. Patients may present with wheeze associated with obstruction of the large airways. Fibre optic bronchoscopy may be needed to investigate the area. Interventional techniques may be needed to alleviate the symptoms.

RESPIRATORY FAILURE

This may be acute or late stage and occur as a result of extensive lung damage in the disease.

LATE COMPLICATIONS

1. Bronchiectasis may be a late complication of pulmonary TB and is caused by extensive lung destruction especially following lobar collapse leading to bronchiectasis. This usually results in chronic copious

long-term sputum production with frequent infective exacerbations. Postural drainage and physiotherapy are often helpful. Prophylactic antibiotics may also be of use.

2. Long-term fibrosis with lung and mediastinal distortion may take place after extensive disease. The trachea may be deviated and infections arise in the area of fibrosis.

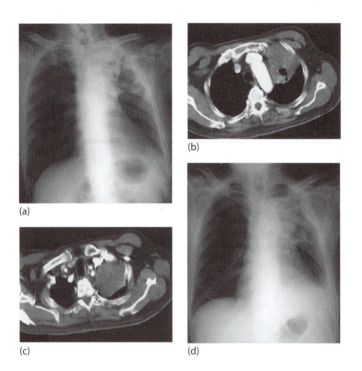

Figure 3.8 Radiological investigation of a 78-year-old man with a 6-week history of productive cough, fever, left-sided chest pain, dyspnoea on exertion and hoarse voice. (a) Chest x-ray and (b) CT scan showed (c) a soft tissue mass in the left upper lobe that encased the left upper lobe bronchus. (d) A chest x-ray performed at the end of TB treatment showed a significant resolution of the initial consolidation seen in the left upper lobe, persistence of the mass (diagnosed as being carcinoid tumour), left upper lobe fibrosis, loss of left lung volume, a left pleural effusion and a large heart shadow.

3. Sometimes a cavity may remain, usually in an upper lobe. This may become colonised with a fungus ball. Sometimes severe haemoptysis may occur requiring resection of the lobe or embolisation (Figure 3.8).

SUMMARY

1. Pulmonary TB is the result of an infection involving any aspect of the respiratory system, i.e. lung parenchyma, pleura, lymph nodes or large airways.
2. A thorough history is important, but there is no specific feature found in the history that helps in diagnosing pulmonary TB.
3. The respiratory examination may be entirely normal.
4. Conformation of diagnosis requires microbiological investigations which may be performed on sputum, bronchoalveolar lavage, pleural fluid, pleural tissue, lymph nodes or parenchymal lung samples.
5. Complications of pulmonary TB can be early, e.g. pneumothorax, or late, e.g. bronchiectasis.
6. Radiographic tests are most commonly chest radiographs and CT scans. Newer modalities such as PET scanning are still under evaluation.
7. The differential diagnosis for pulmonary TB is wide and is dependent on the anatomical area of the respiratory system which is affected.

FURTHER READING

Andreu J, Cáceres J, Pallisa E, Martinez-Rodriguez M. Radiological manifestations of pulmonary tuberculosis. *Eur J Radiol* 2004 Aug;51(2):139–149.

Davies PDO, Gordon GB, Davies G. *Clinical Tuberculosis*, 5th edn. CRC Press, Boca Raton, FL, 2014.

Dugid JP. The numbers and the sites of origin of the droplets expelled during expiratory activities. *Edinb Med J* 1945 Nov;52:385–401.

Kamboj M, Sepkowitz KA. The risk of tuberculosis in patients with cancer. *Clin Infect Dis* 2006 Jun 1;42(11):1592–1595.

Lawn SD, Zumla AI. Tuberculosis. *Lancet* 2011 Jul 2;378(9785):57–72.

Lee CH, Kim K, Hyun MK, Jang EJ, Lee NR, Yim JJ. Use of inhaled corticosteroids and the risk of tuberculosis. *Thorax* 2013 Dec;68(12):1105–1113.

Light RW. Pleural effusions. *Med Clin North Am* 2011 Nov;95(6):1055–1070.

Lois M, Noppen M. Bronchopleural fistulas: An overview of the problem with special focus on endoscopic management. *Chest* 2005 Dec;128(6):3955–3965.

Menzies D, Nahid P. Update in tuberculosis and nontuberculous mycobacterial disease. *Am J Respir Crit Care Med* 2013 Oct 15;188(8):923–927.

Ruderman EM. Overview of safety of non-biologic and biologic DMARDs. *Rheumatology (Oxford)* 2012 Dec;51 Suppl. 6:vi37–vi43.

Sathekge M, Maes A, Kgomo M, Stoltz A, Van de Wiele C. Use of 18F-FDG PET to predict response to first-line tuberculostatics in HIV-associated tuberculosis. *J Nucl Med* 2011 Jun;52(6):880–885.

Sharma SK, Mohan A, Sharma A, Mitra DK. Miliary tuberculosis: New insights into an old disease. *Lancet Infect Dis* 2005 Jul;5(7):415–430.

Vargas D, García L, Gilman RH, Evans C, Ticona E, Navincopa M, Luo RF, Caviedes L, Hong C, Escombe R, Moore DA. Diagnosis of sputum-scarce HIV-associated pulmonary tuberculosis in Lima, Peru. *Lancet* 2005 Jan 8–14;365(9454):150–152.

Wu CY, Hu HY, Pu CY, Huang N, Shen HC, Li CP, Chou YJ. Pulmonary tuberculosis increases the risk of lung cancer: A population-based cohort study. *Cancer* 2011 Feb 1;117(3):618–624.

Zumla A, Raviglione M, Hafner R, von Reyn CF. Tuberculosis. *N Engl J Med* 2013 Feb 21;368(8):745–755.

4

Extra-pulmonary disease

GURINDER TACK AND LAURA WATKINS

EXTRA-PULMONARY SITES OF DISEASE IN TUBERCULOSIS INFECTION

1. Extra-pulmonary tuberculosis (EPTB) refers to disease outside the lungs. However, it often co-exists with pulmonary TB.
2. In the United Kingdom, EPTB accounted for 47% of cases of TB in 2010.
3. Patients with EPTB tend to be slightly younger than patients with pulmonary disease alone.
4. Groups at highest risk of extra-pulmonary disease are health-care workers and, in the western world, foreign-born nationals (especially from the Asian subcontinent).

5. EPTB has known association with HIV co-infection.
6. Outside the lungs, the disease most commonly occurs in peripheral lymph nodes followed by bone and joint infections.
7. EPTB presents a diagnostic challenge, and level of suspicions will often direct a clinician towards starting treatment. Rates of positive TB culture are lower in EPTB at 47% compared to 68% in pulmonary TB alone.

Case study 4.1

FD is a 37-year-old lady who was born in India but had lived in the United Kingdom for 10 years with her husband and two young children. She had noticed a painless swelling on the right side of her neck for 2 months but had no systemic symptoms. She had never had a BCG vaccination, and her maternal grandmother was treated for TB in India when she was a child. FD currently worked as a care assistant in a nursing home. Her GP referred her to an ENT clinic under the 2-week rule for suspected cancer diagnosis in the United Kingdom. The ENT surgeon found several firm, non-tender palpable lymph nodes in the right cervical chain. Subsequent ultrasound investigations of her neck confirmed a 3 cm lymphadenopathy with surrounding oedema. Her surgeon arranged for a CT neck, thorax, abdomen and pelvis and excision of the largest and most accessible node. The CT showed marked right-sided cervical lymphadenopathy and bilateral apical lung fibrosis. Histology of the node showed granuloma formation and positive acid-fast bacilli (AFB) confirmed as *Mycobacterium tuberculosis* on PCR. FD was referred to a respiratory physician who performed an HIV test and commenced quadruple anti-tuberculous treatment immediately.

PERIPHERAL LYMPH NODE TUBERCULOSIS

EPIDEMIOLOGY AND RISK FACTORS

1. Tuberculous lymphadenitis is the most common form of EPTB. Cervical lymph nodes are most frequently involved followed by supraclavicular, mediastinal, axillary and inguinal lymph nodes.
2. Unlike other forms of EPTB, it has a relatively low mortality rate.
3. Women are affected more than men in a ratio of 1.4:1, and it tends to occur in the fourth to fifth decade.

4. Risk factors include patients who are foreign born especially from East Asia, health-care workers and the immunocompromised, particularly those with HIV co-infection.

SYMPTOMS

1. Gradual lymph node enlargement over a 2–3-month period (Figure 4.1).
2. Patients can also report constitutional symptoms such as night sweats, weight loss or fatigue.
3. Symptoms of respiratory TB may be present.

INVESTIGATIONS

1. It is important to investigate thoroughly if there is a high clinical suspicion especially in patients with risk factors. Every effort must be made to exclude co-existing PTB and a chest radiograph should be performed.

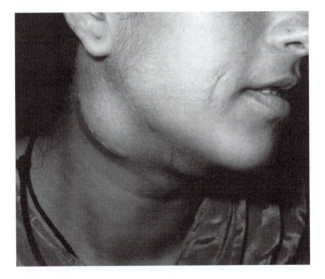

Figure 4.1 Cervical lymphadenopathy in an Asian female present for 3 months; biopsied as no pus on aspiration. Caseating granulomas on histology and *M. tuberculosis* cultured from biopsy material.

2. Ultrasound imaging of lymph nodes reveals hypoechoic change with clear delineation from surrounding tissue. There is often marked surrounding soft tissue oedema.

3. CT also shows peripheral enhancement and a multilocular appearance. Radiologically, they can be differentiated from lymphoma by their heterogenous appearance.

4. The gold standard for diagnosis needs tissue conformation. Lymph node excision is preferred to fine-needle aspiration (FNA), and this reveals a sensitivity of up to 80%.

DIAGNOSIS

1. Diagnosis is confirmed by culturing mycobacterium, as with pulmonary TB; not all culture-positive specimens will be AFB positive.

2. Histologically, lymph nodes contain
   a. Multinucleated giant cells
   b. Caseation
   c. Non-specific lymphoid infiltrates
   d. Langerhans giant cells

TREATMENT

1. A standard 6-month treatment regimen of rifampicin and isoniazid with the first 2 months supplemented with pyrazinamide and ethambutol is recommended. There is no current evidence to suggest that longer treatment improves cure rates or reduces relapse rates.

2. Patients must complete treatment even if the lymph node has been completely excised. Treatment should be stopped at the end of 6 months even if new lymph nodes appear or a sinus forms.

3. Lymph nodes can initially enlarge with treatment and often the disease response may be slower than when treating pulmonary TB.

COMPLICATIONS

These include worsening symptoms during treatment (more common in those who are HIV positive), development of new nodes, sinus formation, fistula and development of chylothorax.

Case study 4.2

AL is a 58-year-old gentleman with type 2 diabetes who rarely visited his GP. Over the past few months, his district nurse, who visited to administer daily insulin injections, had become increasingly concerned. She noted AL was becoming increasingly drowsy and confused when she visited. On one occasion, he seemed to be unable to direct his gaze towards her and she informed the GP who visited him at home. An emergency hospital admission was arranged. Whilst reviewing AL, the emergency doctor read his old notes and noted that he had been previously treated for pulmonary TB aged 20. A CT brain was performed which showed cortical atrophy. The following day a lumbar puncture was performed and the CSF appeared slightly turbid. Treatment for bacterial meningitis was therefore initiated. However, CSF results showed a high lymphocyte count and negative gram stain. A second lumbar puncture was performed and 6 mL of CSF obtained for AFB and TB culture. Anti-tuberculous treatment was started whilst the results were awaited. The CSF subsequently showed acid-fast bacilli and the TB culture later became positive.

TUBERCULOSIS OF THE CENTRAL NERVOUS SYSTEM

EPIDEMIOLOGY AND RISK FACTORS

1. There are only around 100 new cases of neurological TB diagnosed in England and Wales each year.
2. It has a high mortality and morbidity rate. It is invariably due to TB elsewhere in the body. The blood borne spread from pulmonary infection forms subpial and subependymal foci that may later rupture causing meningitis or forming a tuberculoma without meningitis (Figure 4.2).
3. Patients with miliary disease are at highest risk of neurological TB.
4. In developing countries, young children are mostly affected; however, in the United Kingdom, adults, often immigrants, account for most cases.
5. The risk factors of neurological TB are similar to that of lymph node TB, particularly
   a. Immunocompromised, especially with HIV co-infection
   b. Born in or lived in a high prevalence country
   c. Contact with cases of pulmonary TB

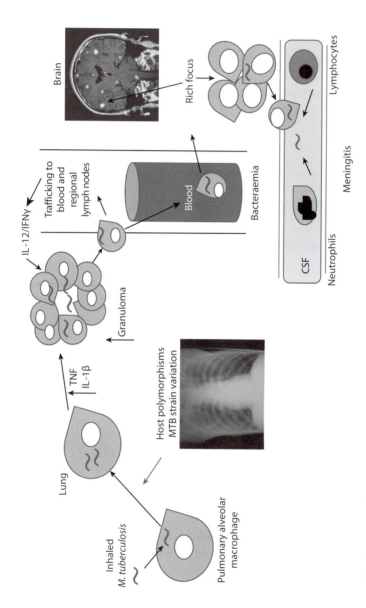

Figure 4.2 Summary of CNS tuberculosis pathogenesis.

SYMPTOMS

1. Insidious onset of vague symptoms over 2–6 weeks means early diagnosis can be difficult. Untreated disease is fatal (Figure 4.3).
2. Headache, fever and vomiting are often present in children; in adults behavioural change such as irritability or apathy may be present. Focal neurological symptoms can develop such as cranial nerve palsies, commonly the sixth, hemiparesis and even seizures.
3. There are three recognised stages of meningitis:

   Stage I.   Conscious, with or without signs of meningeal irritation, no focal neurological deficit

   Stage II. Reduced conscious level and/or focal neurological deficit

   Stage III. Coma
4. Patients with a tuberculoma without meningitis develop features depending on the location of the lesion.
5. Frequently, there are no symptoms; however, some do develop constitutional symptoms and even seizures.

Time (weeks)		0	1	2	3	4	5	
Clinical	Fatigue	+	++	++	++	++	++	D
	Fever	±	+	+	+	+	+	e
	Headache	±	+	++	++	++	++	a
	Consciousness			↓	↓↓	↓↓↓	↓↓↓	t
	Focal signs			+	++	++	++	h
	MRC grade	I	I	II	II/III	III	III	
CSF	White cells		↑ Neutrophils	↑ Neutrophils	↑	↑	↑	
	Protein	↑	↑	↑↑	↑↑	↑↑	↑↑	
	Glucose		↓	↓	↓↓	↓↓	↓↓↓	
	Lactate		↑	↑	↑↑	↑↑	↑↑↑	
	Bacteria		+	+	+	++	++	
Brain imaging	Hydrocephalus		+	++	+++	+++	+++	
	Infarction			+	++	++	++	
	Tuberculoma				+	+	++	
Mortality		5%	10%	20%	30%	50%	80%	
Time (weeks)		0	1	2	3	4	5	

Figure 4.3 Natural history and clinical features of untreated TB meningitis.

INVESTIGATIONS

1. Baseline investigations include
   a. Bloods including full blood count, renal function, liver function, glucose, CRP and ESR
   b. Blood cultures
   c. Chest radiograph
   d. CT brain with contrast, or MRI brain
   e. Lumbar puncture (LP)
   f. HIV test
2. The chest radiograph is abnormal in up to 50% of patients. Every patient with suspected tuberculous meningitis should have a contrast enhanced CT brain as part of routine investigations if available. This should be done within 48 hours after the treatment is started.
3. The CT brain can be normal in elderly patients.
4. Common abnormal findings are hydrocephalus and basal contrast enhancing exudates. Tuberculomas appear as contrast enhancing ring lesions with surrounding oedema (Figure 4.4).
5. An LP is essential. If the initial LP is normal but clinical suspicion remains higher, the LP should be repeated within 48 hours. At least 6 mL of CSF is needed for microbiology to perform Ziehl–Neelsen stain for AFB, TB culture and PCR testing for mycobacterium DNA. The sample should also be sent for analysis of glucose and protein and to culture tests such as AFB and TB culture, and a PCR should be performed to check the presence of mycobacterium. HIV-positive patients should also have CSF tested for *Cryptococcus*.
6. The typical CSF changes are shown in Table 4.1.
7. The opening pressure can be high (>25 cm H_2O in 50%).

DIAGNOSIS

1. AFB in CSF is seen in up to 80% and increased volume of CSF increases diagnostic yield. CSF is less likely to be positive for AFB/culture in patients with tuberculomas, and brain biopsy should be performed for diagnosis (unless there is another site of disease more amenable to sampling).
2. Use of tuberculin skin testing and interferon gamma release assays are of limited use and can often be negative in patients with neurological TB.

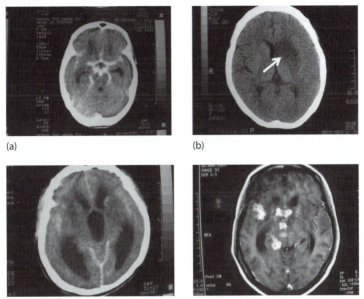

(a)

(b)

(c)

(d)

Figure 4.4 Pathological features of TBM revealed by brain imaging. (a) CT brain post-contrast showing intense enhancement of basal meningeal exudates, typical of TBM. (b) CT brain without contrast showing large infarct in the territory of the middle cerebral artery associated with TBM. (c) CT brain post-contrast showing severe hydrocephalus secondary to TBM. (d) T1-weighted MRI post-contrast showing numerous enhancing and coalescing tuberculomas 8 weeks into the treatment of TBM.

Table 4.1 CSF changes in TB vs. bacterial meningitis

	Protein	Glucose	Cell count	Culture
TB meningitis	Raised	Low CSF: blood <0.5	Leucocytosis Lymphocyte rich	AFB, TB culture, PCR for MTB DNA
Bacterial meningitis	Normal to raised	Low CSF: blood <0.5	Leucocytosis Polymorph rich	Gram stain positive

TREATMENT

1. Treatment is recommended for 12 months.
2. An important consideration is whether the drug will penetrate the blood–brain barrier. Ethionamide, isoniazid, prothionamide and pyrazinamide achieve best penetration. Rifampicin penetrates less and ethambutol and streptomycin are only effective if the meninges are inflamed.
3. The duration of recommended treatment is 12 months: an initial 2 months of rifampicin, isoniazid, pyrazinamide and usually ethambutol, then complete with isoniazid and rifampicin.
4. Steroids are currently recommended by the UK body NICE, although the evidence is not clear cut. Doses are 20–40 mg if on rifampicin, otherwise 10–20 mg/day. The steroid dose should be tapered 2–3 weeks after initiation of treatment.
5. The neurological condition can deteriorate on treatment due to infarction, hydrocephalus and expansion of tuberculomas. Hyponatraemia can develop with associated worsening neurological function; the mechanism is not clear and definitive treatment unclear.

BONE AND JOINT TUBERCULOSIS

EPIDEMIOLOGY AND RISK FACTORS

1. Bone and joint TB presents 3–5 years after the initial respiratory infection. Any bone or joint may be affected but the spine is the most common site, accounting for approximately half of all cases (Figure 4.5).
2. Typically, the thoracic and thoracolumbar spine is involved. Spinal TB can be challenging to diagnose, as the symptoms are insidious. Spinal infection starts in the intervertebral discs causing a discitis. This spreads along the spinal ligaments to the adjacent vertebrae resulting in loss of disc space.
3. As the disease progresses, there is destruction of the vertebrae and loss of vertebral height causing kyphosis. Multiple levels of the spine can also be involved.

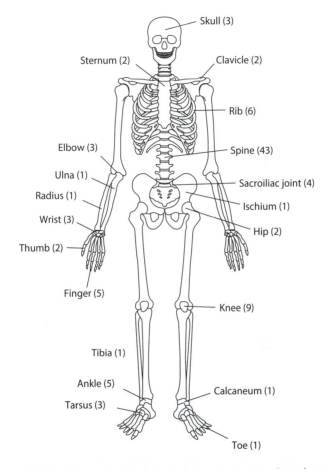

Figure 4.5 Sites of bony tuberculosis in Asian patients. Number of patients for each site in parentheses. (From Hodgson SP and Ormerod LP, *J R Coll Surg Edinb*, 35, 259, 1990.)

Symptoms

1. The most common symptom of spinal TB is back pain (can present weeks or months before diagnosis), local tenderness and progressive kyphosis.
2. Other presentations may include motor and sensory symptoms due to spinal cord compression leading to paraplegia (Pott's paraplegia).
3. Spinal TB may also be complicated by abscesses suggested by a para-spinal mass or a psoas abscess formation.

Diagnosis

1. The diagnosis may be delayed due to low prevalence and insidious nature of the disease. In endemic areas, diagnosis is mainly by using x-rays, showing loss of the vertebral cortex (Figure 4.6).

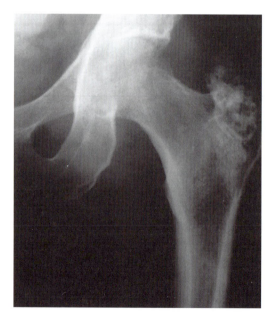

Figure 4.6 Tuberculosis of the left hip and greater trochanter presenting with a sinus over the hip from which *M. tuberculosis* was isolated.

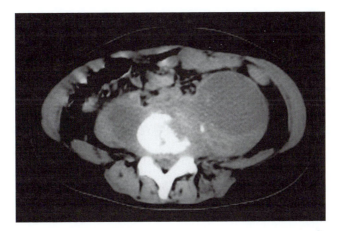

Figure 4.7 Bilateral L > R psoas abscesses related to spinal disease. Presented with left psoas spasm. One litre of pus drained from left by ultrasound-guided aspiration, which grew *M. tuberculosis.*

2. In developed countries, advancements in scanning techniques such as CT and MRI have improved the diagnosis of spinal TB. Changes may appear on scan even before they are seen on plain x-rays.
3. The features of spine TB are that of para-spinal shadow in the thoracic spine indicating the presence of an abscess. Differential diagnosis includes metastatic disease and pyogenic infection (Figure 4.7).
4. The diagnosis is confirmed with an open/needle biopsy of the spinal lesion. It is important to take appropriate cultures for mycobacterial disease in addition to pyogenic infections, to avoid delayed diagnosis and treatment.

TREATMENT

1. Treatment is similar to that of pulmonary disease. Current American Thoracic Society and Centers for Disease Control and Prevention guidelines recommend 6 months treatment for spinal TB unless there is central nervous system involvement.
2. The role of surgery in spinal TB remains controversial. Patients with spinal disease without instability or evidence of spinal cord compression should be treated medically. Only those with spinal instability or

spinal cord compression should be considered for anterior spinal fusion surgery.

3. A recent Cochrane study from a 2010 review found no difference between chemotherapy and surgery versus chemotherapy alone. However the authors did conclude that clinicians may judge that surgery may be indicated in subgroups of patients such as those with an initial kyphosis angle greater than 30° (especially in children) or progressive or persistent neurological deficit with spinal cord compression despite chemotherapy.

4. Although the spine is the commonest site of infection, any bone or joint can be affected. Other sites of involvement may include hip, knee or elbow joint, or the bones of the hand or foot. TB osteomyelitis may also develop. Treatment involves standard therapy and input from the orthopaedic team.

PERICARDIAL TUBERCULOSIS

PATHOGENESIS OF DISEASE

1. Pericardial disease due to TB (which can result in acute pericarditis, constrictive pericarditis or tamponade) accounts for 4%–7% of cases in the developing countries. Pericardial TB usually results from the direct spread of infection from mediastinal glands, although occasionally spread may be haematogenous.

2. Acute pericarditis is caused by an immune response to tuberculous proteins and an exudative pericardial effusion can result. This can progress to chronic pericarditis with granulomatous inflammation, leading to fibrosis and eventually calcification.

SYMPTOMS

1. The symptoms of tuberculous pericarditis are insidious, non-specific and similar to other forms of TB. Symptoms include
   a. Fever
   b. Malaise
   c. Night sweats
   d. Weight loss

    e. Cough

    f. Chest pain

    g. Breathlessness

    h. Orthopnoea

2. Clinical findings of pericardial TB may include fever, increased jugular venous pressure (JVP), tachycardia, pleural dullness and peripheral oedema. There may also be a pericardia rub, quiet heart sounds, ascites and hepatomegaly. Clinical findings depend on the stage of pericardial involvement.

3. In constrictive pericarditis, signs include quiet heart sounds, raised JVP, pulsus paradoxus, peripheral oedema, abdominal distension, dyspnoea and a venous pressure which rises with inspiration (Kussmaul's sign).

4. If the pericardial effusion is large enough, cardiac tamponade may develop with signs of low blood pressure, narrow pulse pressure, tachycardia, raised JVP and prominent pulsus paradoxus.

DIAGNOSIS

1. Pericardial TB should be suspected in patients from endemic areas who present with a fever, pericardial effusion or signs of tamponade.

2. Chest x-ray usually reveals cardiomegaly and a pleural effusion. Calcification may be present in chronic pericarditis. Associated pulmonary TB may be seen in up to 30% of patients and sputum smear and culture should be done. The tuberculin test is usually positive in 80%–100% of patients with TB.

3. There are no specific ECG changes in pericardial TB; however, small QRS complexes and generalised T-wave changes may be seen in effusions. Echocardiogram is the best way of confirming the presence of a pericardial effusion. Pericardial thickening may also be seen. Cardiac tamponade may reveal compression of right heart and in constrictive pericarditis there will be thickening of the pericardium. In resource-rich settings, MRI and CT can also be used.

4. Pericardiocentesis is often required to confirm the diagnosis and can also provide therapeutic relief of symptoms. The fluid is an exudate (protein >35 g/L) and is usually lymphocytic but polymorphs can be present in early disease. Diagnosis is confirmed by the presence of AFB in the fluid. Pericardial biopsy can also be done and show granulomatous histology on biopsy.

Treatment

1. For patients with active pericardial TB, treatment should be the standard recommended regimen. Some studies have shown that treatment with isoniazid/rifampicin for 6 months supplemented by streptomycin and pyrazinamide for 3 months worked for both constriction and effusion.
2. The role of steroids may reduce the requirement for open drainage and repeated pericardiocentesis. Therefore, for adults, a glucocorticoid equivalent to prednisolone at 60 mg/day should be considered as part of initial treatment with gradual tapering of the dose within 2–3 weeks.
3. There is conflicting evidence about the role of surgery. It should be reserved for those with late presentations and life-threatening tamponade or for those who fail medical treatment.

GENITOURINARY TUBERCULOSIS

Epidemiology and risk factors

1. Genitourinary tuberculosis (GUTB) occurs in approximately 3%–4% of patients with pulmonary TB and is common in the first few months of primary infection.
2. However, clinical disease can also develop up to 20 years later, as the organism lays dormant in the renal parenchyma.

Symptoms

1. GUTB is often a silent disease, which progresses insidiously. TB tubercles are formed in kidneys, and the lesions usually heal spontaneously. However, they may enlarge and rupture leading to complete unilateral renal destruction before diagnosis is even made.
2. Constitutional symptoms of fever, weight loss and night sweats are common. As the disease progresses patients may present with dysuria, haematuria, sterile pyuria, flank pain, renal mass and recurrent urinary tract infections.
3. Renal disease can spread to the ureters causing stenosis with obstructive uropathy and to the bladder causing inflammation and fibrosis.

DIAGNOSIS

1. Typically, GUTB is positive for haematuria and proteinuria on dipstick. There may be pus cells seen on microscopy but culture is negative for bacterial pathogens-sterile pyuria.
2. Ultrasound may show hydronephrosis and small kidneys but is not specific. CT scanning may show calcification and give further information about the renal tract. For urinary tract TB, an intravenous pyelogram (IVP) may be useful.
3. In all patients with suspected GUTB, three early morning urines should be sent for TB culture. In some instances, surgery may be required to obtain tissue for culture.

TREATMENT

Surgery may be appropriate but all patients with GUTB should complete the standard recommended chemotherapy regimen.

ABDOMINAL TUBERCULOSIS

PATHOGENESIS OF DISEASE

1. Abdominal TB encompasses disease of the intestinal tract (any site can be affected; the ileocaecal area is the most common site due to the high concentration of lymphoid tissues in this area), peritoneum, omentum and the solid intra-abdominal organs.
2. It can occur due to the reactivation of foci in the abdomen from a primary PTB infection, ingestion of infected sputum, haematogenous spread from other sites or contiguous spread from genitourinary TB.
3. Risk factors include
   a. Liver cirrhosis
   b. HIV co-infection
   c. Diabetes
   d. Malignancy
   e. Use of anti-TNF agents
   f. Continuous ambulatory peritoneal dialysis

Symptoms

1. One-third of patients present acutely with abdominal pain, usually the right iliac fossa (RIF), or bowel obstruction. The other two-thirds have an insidious onset with fever, malaise, weight loss and abdominal pain being prominent symptoms.
2. Peritoneal TB can present with ascites, adhesions or omental thickening and fibrosis which can result in loculated ascites.

Investigations

1. Investigations to examine the gastrointestinal tract include
   a. Small bowel barium meal or follow through
   b. Barium enema
   c. CT
   d. Ultrasound
   e. Endoscopy
2. The ileocaecal valve is often incompetent (in contrast to Crohn's disease) and this can be identified on barium imaging. Barium studies can also reveal strictures (Figures 4.8 and 4.9).
3. Ultrasound imaging can show enlarged heterogenous lymph nodes. It is also used to identify ascites and its position for aspiration. The caecum can be shrunken and displaced out of the RIF on CT imaging due to mesenteric fibrosis.
4. CT also identifies other areas of abnormality in the bowel and peritoneum.
5. Endoscopically, ulcers in large bowel are confluent and superficial and they mostly do not penetrate the muscularis. As ulcers heal, strictures form.
6. Laparoscopy is considered if the diagnosis is still not clear or tissue cannot be obtained via other methods. It enables visualisation of the omentum and peritoneum to look for tubercles and thickening. Biopsies of macroscopically abnormal areas can be taken.

Diagnosis

1. Diagnosis is confirmed with histology (granulomas or caseating necrosis) or microbiology (AFB or culture positive).
2. Histology of colonic biopsy has a lower yield as the inflammation is submucosal and may not be included in the biopsy.

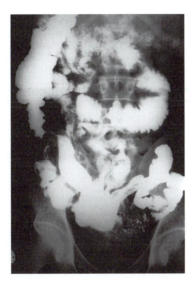

Figure 4.8 Tuberculosis of the small bowel and caecum. Barium follow-through showing strictures in the ileum and at the ileocaecal junction with an abnormal lower pole of the caecum.

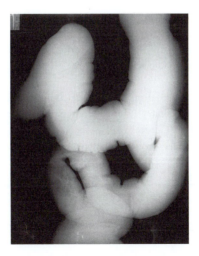

Figure 4.9 Barium enema in a 38-year-old Asian woman with two stone (13 kg) weight loss. Obstruction in the ascending colon is shown mimicking carcinoma. Ileocaecal tuberculosis was resected.

3. Ascitic fluid is proteinaceous and has a high lymphocyte count; the serum ascetic albumin gradient is <1.1. AFB and culture is less likely to be positive.

TREATMENT

Treatment is usually with 6 months of standard anti-tuberculous therapy.

LEARNING POINTS

1. Extra-pulmonary TB presents a diagnostic challenge and level of suspicion will often direct a clinician towards starting treatment.
2. In the United Kingdom, extra-pulmonary TB accounted for 47% of cases of TB in 2010.
3. Tuberculous lymphadenitis is the most common form of extra-pulmonary TB.
4. In developing countries, young children are mostly affected by neurological tuberculosis particularly TB meningitis.
5. Treatment of TB meningitis is with standard TB therapy for 12 months.
6. In bone and joint TB, any bone or joint may be affected but the spine is the most common site, accounting for approximately half of all cases.
7. Pericardial disease due to TB (acute pericarditis, constrictive pericarditis or tamponade) accounts for 4%–7% of cases in developing countries.
8. Genitourinary tuberculosis (GUTB) occurs in approximately 3%–4% of patients with pulmonary TB and is common in the first few months of primary infection. Clinical disease can also develop up to 20 years later, as the organism lays dormant in the renal parenchyma.
9. In abdominal TB, one-third of patients present acutely with abdominal pain, usually the right iliac fossa (RIF), or with bowel obstruction. The other two-thirds have an insidious onset with fever, malaise, weight loss and abdominal pain.
10. With the exception of TB meningitis, most cases of extra-pulmonary present chronically over months.
11. The duration of treatment is 6 months, which is standard, the exception being TB meningitis which is treated for 12 months.

FURTHER READING

Davies PDO, Gordon GB, Davies G. *Clinical Tuberculosis*, 5th edn. CRC Press, Boca Raton, FL, 2014.

Fontanillo JM, Barnes A, Fordham A, von Reyn. Current diagnosis and management of peripheral Tuberculous lymphadenitis. *Clin Infect Dis* 2011;53:555–556.

Hodgson SP, Ormerod LP, Ten-year experience of bone and joint tuberculosis in Blackburn 1978–1987. *JR Coll Surg Edinb* 1990;35(4):259–262.

Jutte PC, van Loenhout-Rooyackers JH. *Routine Surgery in Addition to Chemotherapy for Treating Spinal Tuberculosis Cochrane Infectious* Database Systematic Reviews 2006, Issue 1, Art. No. C0004532. John Wiley & Sons, Ltd., Hoboken, NJ.

National Institute for Health and Clinical Excellence. Tuberculosis: Clinical diagnosis and management of tuberculosis, and measures for its prevention and control. NICE clinical guideline 117. NICE, London, U.K., 2011. https://www.nice.org.uk/guidance/cg117/resources/guidance-tuberculosis-pdf. Accessed August 2015.

Ruslami R et al. Intensified regimen containing rifampicin and moxifloxacin for tuberculous meningitis: An open-label, randomised controlled phase 2 trial. *Lancet Infect Dis* 2013;13:27–35.

Sharma SK, Bhatia V. Abdominal tuberculosis. *Indian J Med Res* October 2004;120(4):305–315.

Sharma SK, Mohan A. Extrapulmonary tuberculosis. *Indian J Med Res* October 2004;120(4):316–353.

Strang JIG. Management of tuberculous constrictive pericarditis and tuberculous pericardial effusion in Transkei: Results at 10 years follow-up. *Q J Med* 2004;97:52535.

Thwaites G, Fisher M, Hemingway C, Scott G, Solomon T, Innes J. British infection society guidelines for the diagnosis and treatment of tuberculosis of the central nervous system in adults and children. *J Infect* 2009;59:167–187.

5

Tuberculosis in children

DAVID KK HO

BACKGROUND

1. The 2012 World Health Organization (WHO) Report estimated the global burden of childhood tuberculosis to be 490,000 cases and deaths to be 64,000 per year.
2. However, accurate estimations of the burden of childhood tuberculosis are difficult to quantify due to a number of factors including inaccurate reporting, difficulties with diagnosing TB in childhood and HIV co-infection.
3. Data on childhood TB incidence are less accurate from high prevalence areas.
4. An increase in incidence of childhood TB may be due to a number of factors including
   a. HIV co-infection
   b. Immigration and travel patterns

    c. Decreasing socioeconomic status in areas of high disease prevalence

    d. Emergence of drug-resistant strains of TB

5. Diagnosis in children can be difficult and require a different strategy to adults:

    a. A history of contact with tuberculosis patients is vital to establish.

    b. Up to 50% of children with active tuberculosis may be asymptomatic in early disease.

    c. A number of scoring systems for diagnosis have been developed but there are no universally accepted methods.

6. Cases of congenital TB have been reported where disease is presumed to have been transmitted *in utero*. The mortality for this is high.

Case study 5.1

AT is a 5-month-old girl who was admitted to the children's ward of her local hospital because of a positive Mantoux test (22 mm) which was read at 48 hours. Her mother had been diagnosed with TB 3 weeks previously and had been commenced on quadruple therapy. At the same time, the girl was commenced on preventative therapy consisting of isoniazid and pyridoxine. AT's family was from Pakistan and they moved to the United Kingdom 18 months ago. AT had been feeding well and was gaining weight. There was no history of fever or weight loss. Her maternal grandmother was diagnosed with TB 6 years ago. Her mother developed a cough 3 weeks into the pregnancy; however, that was not investigated further at the time. The girl was born healthy at term by normal vaginal delivery weighing 3.1 kg. She received a BCG when she was 11 weeks old and had three sets of vaccinations according to the UK immunisation schedule.

On examination she looked well, bright and active. Her head circumference was 39.4 cm (0.4th centile) and her weight was 5.6 kg (2nd centile). She had bilateral vesicular breath sounds with no wheeze and had a respiratory rate of 28. A 1 cm cervical lymphadenopathy was felt on the right side, and she had no axillary, or inguinal lymphadenopathy. She had a soft anterior fontanelle and was neurologically and developmentally appropriate. Her abdomen was soft with liver edge felt 1 cm below the costophrenic angle. A chest radiograph revealed changes consistent with miliary TB. Her blood tests showed lymphocytosis and a mildly raised ESR of 44. Her interferon gamma release assay was positive and her HIV test was negative. Three gastric washings were collected and sent for microscopy and culture. A lumbar puncture was performed which drew clear and colourless fluid. Microscopy revealed WBC <3, RBC 13, with no AFB seen. CSF glucose was 2.8 (serum glucose 4.5) and protein was 0.14. An ultrasound of the abdomen showed extensive lymphadenopathy within the abdomen along the porta-hepatis, celiac trunk and para-aortic region. A CT scan confirmed lymphadenopathy seen additionally in both inguinal areas, with normal appearances of the liver, kidneys, pancreas, spleen and gall bladder.

In view of the findings AT commenced on quadruple therapy. An eye examination by the ophthalmologist was reported to be normal. Whilst on the ward there were concerns regarding vomiting after taking the medications. The timing of the medication was spaced out during the day with good effect. She was discharged home after 1 week.

Her MRI brain was initially reported to be of normal appearance. However, an amendment 18 days later showed focal abnormality in the medial cortex of the left parietal lobe. These appearances were consistent with a tuberculoma. A decision was made not to commence corticosteroids as the patient was clinically well and 4 weeks had lapsed since the start of the treatment.

She was reviewed in the TB clinic at almost 7 months of age. A chest radiograph showed loss of volume on the right side with shift of the mediastinum to the right. A repeat CT scan showed evidence of paratracheal lymphadenopathy, anterior mediastinal and a subcarinal soft tissue mass. The mass was seen compressing the right lower lobe bronchus causing collapse of the right lower lobe particularly the posterior segment. Prednisolone 10 mg was commenced for a month. She was admitted for direct laryngo-tracheo-bronchoscopy. The bronchoscopy showed endotracheal disease and a large cast, which was removed with suction and forceps. Histology showed necrotic material surrounded by a rim of granulomatous inflammation, comprising epithelioid histiocytes, lymphocytes, plasma cells and scattered neutrophils. A Ziehl–Neelsen stain showed small numbers of acid-fast bacilli. Special stains for bacteria and fungi were negative. A chest radiograph immediately after the procedure showed some improvement. At 10 months of age, parents reported improvement in breathing particularly early mornings. Prednisolone was weaned down and stopped after a normal synacthen test 4 months later. The patient completed a year of treatment and was discharged from the clinic at 2 years of age.

HISTORY

There are a number of important questions to ask in regard to the clinical history and these are detailed in the following.

CURRENT SYMPTOMS

1. *Cough*: Unlike adults, many children will not have symptoms when diagnosed with tuberculosis. Pulmonary lesions are the most common form of TB in children. Therefore, TB needs to be considered in children in endemic areas or had history of exposure to TB, who present with a prolonged history of cough.
2. *Sputum*: TB in children is a paucibacillary disease. In addition, children often struggle to provide adequate sputum samples. Induced sputum provides the highest yield compared to other methods of sputum collection. In infants where induced sputum is not possible, gastric washings can be used instead.
3. *Lymph node enlargement*: Following primary infection, local spread of disease results in tuberculosis lymphadenopathy. Lymph nodes can be intrathoracic or extrapulmonary. Extrapulmonary TB is more common in children than adults and often presents with the primary lung lesion in the supraclavicular and paratracheal regions.
4. *Fatigue*: Persistent fatigue has a good diagnostic value in children with suspected tuberculosis. This symptom often disappears when children respond to anti-TB medication.
5. *Weight loss/faltering growth*: In children that are at risk of developing TB, weight loss or faltering growth is a sensitive marker that aids the diagnosis of TB once other causes of weight loss are ruled out. Weight gain is often seen once TB is treated.
6. *Fever and night sweats*: Fever and night sweats are less common in children with tuberculosis. However, persistent and non-remitting nature of fever can help one to distinguish TB from other infections.
7. *Headache and vomiting*: Although headache and vomiting are not specific symptoms to tuberculosis in the central nervous system, one should be alerted to the possibility of disease if a child is at risk of TB. Retrospective case series have shown around 50% of patients with tuberculous meningitis presented with headache and vomiting.

8. *Seizures*: Children who have tuberculous meningitis are much more likely to present with seizure than adults. Case series from London and Turkey both showed more than 50% of children with tuberculous meningitis initially presenting with seizures.

RISK FACTORS

1. *Age*: The risk of developing disease following primary TB infection is approximately 50% in children under 1 year of age; the risk decreases to 20% in those at 1–2 years of age and further decreases to 5% in those at 2–5 years of age. Infants with immature immune systems are at highest risk of developing disseminated disease. Data from the pre-chemotherapy era show that the risk of disease is lowest in children at 5–10 years of age. In the teenage years, the risk of developing disease rises again and children develop adult type of disease.

2. *Immune status*: HIV-infected children are more likely to develop active disease and more severe disease. A study in South Africa showed a 20-fold increase in the incidence of TB in HIV-infected children. Other groups of immunocompromised children include very young children that are on immunosuppression, children undergoing transplant and children with cancer.

3. *Contacts with TB*: History of contact with adults who have TB is important as diagnosis is difficult in children. A significant proportion of children with TB are identified through contact tracing in countries with lower prevalence. The primary area of contact is through their homes; other important areas of contact include school or workplace.

4. *Nutrition*: Children with malnutrition have impaired cell-mediated immunity, and various observational studies show a link between malnutrition and TB. However, faltering growth is one of the symptoms in children with TB, and it can be difficult to know which comes first. Vitamin D deficiency has been shown to be associated with TB in UK immigrants.

5. *Vaccination history*: It is important to ask about the history of Bacille Calmette–Guérin (BCG) vaccination as the majority of current studies show that children who have not been BCG vaccinated are at higher risk of developing pulmonary tuberculosis infection than those who have been vaccinated.

SOCIAL AND FAMILY HISTORY

1. *Genetic susceptibility*: Various genes have been identified through genome-wide studies. In particular, some susceptible genes have been found to implicate more severe disease. These genes are involved in the upregulation of macrophages through the interferon-γ/interleukin-12 pathway.
2. *Social factors*: Poverty is central to all risk factors that increase the likelihood of developing tuberculosis. With poverty comes poor housing and overcrowding, delayed diagnosis and treatment. These factors all contribute to the increased prevalence of TB.

EXAMINATION

1. *General appearance*: Children in endemic areas often present with advanced disease compared to children in areas where TB prevalence is low. Children with advanced disease can present ill looking and with signs of faltering growth. This is in contrast to children presenting without any signs or symptoms in areas where the prevalence is low, where cases are detected through screening.
2. *Clubbing*: Digital clubbing is associated with a number of causes. However, as clubbing is uncommon in children, the presence of clubbing should prompt one to look for TB especially in endemic areas. Studies have shown correlation between digital clubbing and pulmonary TB, which was not affected by human immunodeficiency virus infection.
3. *Examination of the chest*: The pathophysiology of tuberculosis in children is such that it produces different clinical entities.
   a. Focal clinical signs in young children are generally harder to illicit. In children less than 2 years of age, the risk of disseminated disease following primary infection is high.
   b. However, it is not possible to distinguish tuberculosis from other lower respiratory tract infections by examining the chest alone, even if miliary TB is present.
   c. Children less than 5 years of age often have airway complications from lymph nodes disease because the airways are small.

An airway can be compressed either from the outside or from intra-luminal disease. This can then cause atelectasis and collapse or hyperinflation of parts of the lung depending on the extent of the obstruction.

  d. Pleural effusion is more frequently seen in children older than 5 years of age and can indicate recent primary infection.
  e. In post-pubertal children, one can see the adult type of cavitating disease.

4. *Lymph nodes*: A study in South Africa showed that 20% of children with TB have extrapulmonary disease, and of those children with extrapulmonary TB, 50% have peripheral lymphadenopathy. These lymph nodes are firm and non-tender and often grow over a period of time with cervical and supraclavicular regions most frequently affected.

5. *Neurology*: It is important to perform a neurological assessment in children presenting with TB.
  a. In children under 2 years old, the risk of developing tuberculous meningitis is higher than in older children.
  b. Bulging anterior fontanelle and increasing head circumference are useful indicators for meningitis in children whose cranial sutures have not fused.
  c. In older children, stiff neck, positive kerning sign, abnormal GCS or cranial nerve palsies should raise the question of possible tuberculous meningitis.
  d. However, definite diagnosis of tuberculous meningitis requires a lumbar puncture.

6. *Systematic review*: TB can manifest in all parts of the body. Other important areas to be considered in a child who is at risk of TB include the abdomen, bones and joints, skin and eyes.

INVESTIGATIONS

Sputum

1. TB is a paucibacillary disease in children, and getting adequate sample of sputum can be difficult. In addition to obtaining sample, laboratory backup is essential.

2. Young children swallow a significant proportion of sputum, and therefore, gastric lavage when performed on three consecutive mornings has been shown to be more effective than bronchoalveolar lavage in a hospital setting.
3. When comparing gastric lavage to induction of sputum, where children received hypertonic saline first followed by physiotherapy, induction of sputum showed slightly better yield.
4. If performing induction of sputum, one needs to have adequate barrier protection and a room with proper ventilation.
5. Novel techniques like the string test where one swallows a capsule attached to a string and then retrieving it 4 hours later has not been extensively studied in children.

IMAGING

1. Chest radiograph
   a. As pulmonary TB is the most common form of TB and microbiological yield is low, chest radiograph remains an important tool in the diagnosis of TB and monitoring of treatment.
   b. Studies from South Africa have shown a sensitivity of 39% for detecting TB in children using chest radiograph.
   c. Even a low-sensitivity chest radiograph is helpful in differentiating between airspace disease, miliary TB and lymph node disease.
2. Chest computed tomography
   a. Computed tomography (CT) has enabled us to detect lymph node enlargement that is otherwise not seen on chest radiograph.
   b. Studies from South Africa have shown up to 92% of patients with WHO criteria of clinical suspected TB had mediastinal or hilar lymph nodes.
   c. Although there is still no consensus regarding whether these lymph nodes should be considered as active disease or latent TB, it can be useful for diagnosing TB in immunocompromised host (Figure 5.1).
3. Brain imaging
   a. CT is often performed first as it is fast and more readily available (Figure 5.2).
   b. Magnetic resonance imaging (MRI) offers more details; however, it often requires sedation or general anaesthesia as children cannot

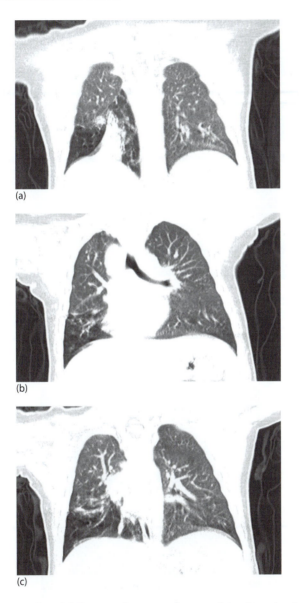

(a)

(b)

(c)

Figure 5.1 (a, b and c) Computed tomography scan of the chest showing collapse of the right lower lobe particularly the posterior segment. There is also shifting of the mediastinum to the right.

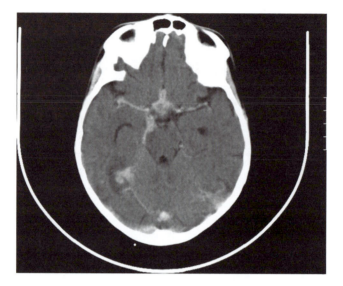

Figure 5.2 Computed tomography scan of the head showing basal enhancement consistent with tuberculous meningitis.

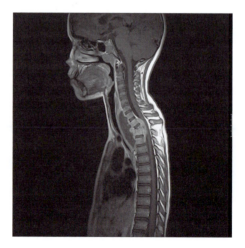

Figure 5.3 Magnetic resonance image showing spinal tuberculosis.

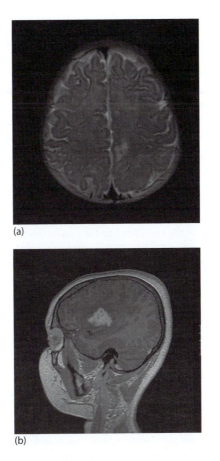

(a)

(b)

Figure 5.4 (a and b) Magnetic resonance images of the brain showing CNS tuberculoma.

        tolerate the long time period required to obtain a scan (Figures 5.3 and 5.4).

c. Brain imaging is performed if one presents with seizures or other neurological symptoms.

d. Tuberculomas can be seen with or without meningitis on both modes of imaging.

e. Meningitis classically shows basal enhancement with or without infarcts and hydrocephalus.

IMMUNE-BASED DIAGNOSTICS

1. Tuberculin skin test
   a. The tuberculin skin test (TST) involves injection of a purified protein derivative intradermally and after 48 hours, measuring the size of the reaction.
   b. The sensitivity and specificity of TST was 80% and 85% from recent systematic review and meta-analyses, which were similar to the newer serum immune-based diagnostic methods.
   c. However, the sensitivity of the TST decreases in children of younger age and in HIV-infected children. False-positive results have been a concern with neonatal BCG vaccination.
   d. Studies have shown that 4 years after the neonatal BCG, there is no difference in the vaccinated and the unvaccinated groups if 10 mm is used as a cut-off point. TST results of greater than 15 mm were more likely due to TB infection.
2. Interferon γ release assays
   a. There are two IGRAs that are available commercially: the Quanti-FERON-TB Gold In-Tube assay (QFT; Cellestis/Qiagen Carnegie, Australia) and the T-SPOT.*TB* assay (T-SPOT; Oxford Immunotec, Abingdon, UK). The sensitivity of IGRA is similar to that of TST.
   b. The specificity of IGRA appears to be greater compared to TST and is a useful screening tool in contact tracing in schools or communities. Using both IGRA and TST can lead to improved sensitivity. See the latent TB chapter for further details.
3. Blood tests
   a. Routine blood tests often include a full blood count to look for anaemia. Liver function test is performed as most anti-TB medications can affect liver function.
   b. Urea and creatinine are also performed to assess renal function. Low serum vitamin D levels are associated with higher risk of active TB.
   c. Supplementation with vitamin D may improve host immunity to mycobacteria; however, there is no evidence of clinical benefits.

TREATMENT

1. Drug treatment and duration vary depending on whether TB is active or latent, the site of the disease and the age of the patient.

2. Robust pharmacokinetic and pharmacodynamic data for TB drugs in the paediatric population are lacking.
3. Generally, infants metabolise drugs faster and require a higher dose of drug per kilogram than older children. Multidrug-resistant (MDR) TB and extensively drug-resistant (XDR) TB are rare in children but need to be considered in regions of high prevalence.
4. Table 5.1 details the first-line drugs used in childhood TB. Table 5.2 details specific regimens based on the site of disease.

Table 5.1 Recommended daily dosages of anti-tuberculous drugs for children

Drugs	NICE TB Guidelines (as in BNFC) (United Kingdom)	American Academy of Pediatrics (United States)	World Health Organization
Isoniazid	10 mg/kg max. 300 mg	10–15 mg/kg	10 mg/kg (range 10–15 mg/kg) max. 300 mg per day
Rifampicin	15 mg/kg OD max. 450 mg if body weight <50 kg; max. 600 mg if body weight >50 kg	10–20 mg/kg	15 mg/kg (range 10–20 mg/kg) max. 600 mg per day
Pyrazinamide	35 mg/kg OD max. 1.5 g if body weight <50 kg; max 2 g if body weight >50 kg	30–40 mg/kg	35 mg/kg (range 30–40 mg/kg)
Ethambutol	20 mg/kg OD	20 mg/kg	20 mg/kg (range 15–25 mg/kg)

Sources: National Institute for Health and Clinical Excellence, Tuberculosis: Clinical diagnosis and management of tuberculosis, and measures for its prevention and control. NICE clinical guideline 117, NICE, London, U.K., 2011, https://www.nice.org.uk/guidance/cg117/resources/guidance-tuberculosis-pdf, accessed August 2015; Pickering L et al., *Red Book: 2012 Report of the Committee on Infectious Diseases*, American Academy of Pediatrics, Elk Grove Village, IL, 2012; World Health Organization, *Rapid Advice. Treatment of Tuberculosis in Children*, WHO, Geneva, Switzerland, 2010.

Table 5.2 Recommended treatment schedules for tuberculosis in children

	NICE Guidelines (United Kingdom)	American Academy of Pediatrics	World Health Organization
Drug-susceptible pulmonary TB[a] and extra-pulmonary TB[b]	2 months of RHZE, then 4 months of RH	2 months of R[c]HZ(E[d]), then 4 months of RH	2 months of RHZ[e](E[f]), then 4 months of RH
TB meningitis	2 months of RHZE, then 10 months of RH	2 months of RHZE[g], then 7–10 months of RH	2 months of RHZ, then 10 months of RH
Osteoarticular TB	2 months of RHZE, then 4 months of RH	2 months of RHZE, then 4 months of RH	2 months of RHZE, then 10 months of RH

Sources: National Institute for Health and Clinical Excellence, Tuberculosis: Clinical diagnosis and management of tuberculosis, and measures for its prevention and control. NICE clinical guideline 117, NICE, London, U.K., 2011, https://www.nice.org.uk/guidance/cg117/resources/guidance-tuberculosis-pdf, accessed *August 2015*; Pickering L et al., *Red Book: 2012 Report of the Committee on Infectious Diseases*, American Academy of Pediatrics, Elk Grove Village, IL, 2012; World Health Organization, *Rapid Advice. Treatment of Tuberculosis in Children*, WHO, Geneva, Switzerland, 2010.

Note: R, rifampicin; E, ethambutol; H, isoniazid; S, streptomycin; Z, pyrazinamide.

[a] In the absence of lung cavities.
[b] In both HIV-positive and HIV-negative children.
[c] Rifabutin can be substituted for Rifampacin if there are issues with antiretroviral interaction.
[d] If resistance suspected and can be discontinued once drug resistance is excluded.
[e] In the setting of low HIV prevalence and low isoniazid resistance.
[f] In the setting of high HIV prevalence and high isoniazid resistance or in children with extensive pulmonary disease in the setting of low HIV prevalence and low isoniazid resistance.
[g] Can be substituted with ethionamide or aminoglycoside.

SUMMARY

1. Infants are most at risk for developing disseminated TB including TB meningitis, a diagnosis that carries significant mortality and morbidity.
2. Children are more likely to develop disease after exposure to TB, therefore, almost all children are offered treatment for latent TB.

3. Childhood TB can be very difficult to diagnose but there are no universally accepted diagnostic methods for doing so.
4. The drugs used for treatment in children are generally the same as in cases of adult TB but has to be dosed carefully according to the weight of the children.

FURTHER READING

Abadco DL, Steiner P. Gastric lavage is better than bronchoalveolar lavage for isolation of *Mycobacterium tuberculosis* in childhood pulmonary tuberculosis. *Pediatr Infect Dis J* 1992;11(9):735–738.

Adetifa IM et al. Commercial interferon gamma release assays compared to the tuberculin skin test for diagnosis of latent *Mycobacterium tuberculosis* infection in childhood contacts in the Gambia. *Pediatr Infect Dis J* 2010;29(5):439–443.

Andronikou S, Wieselthaler, N. Modern imaging of tuberculosis in children: Thoracic, central nervous system and abdominal tuberculosis. *Pediatr Radiol* 2004;34(11):861–875.

Andronikou S et al. CT scanning for the detection of tuberculous mediastinal and hilar lymphadenopathy in children. *Pediatr Radiol* 2004;34(3): 232–236.

Chow F et al. La cuerda dulce – A tolerability and acceptability study of a novel approach to specimen collection for diagnosis of paediatric pulmonary tuberculosis. *BMC Infect Dis* 2006;6(1):67.

Cruz AT, Ong LT, Starke JR. Emergency department presentation of children with tuberculosis. *Acad Emerg Med* 2011;18(7):726–732.

Ddungu H, Johnson JL, Smieja M, Mayanja-Kizza H. Digital clubbing in tuberculosis–relationship to HIV infection, extent of disease and hypo-albuminemia. *BMC infectious diseases.* 2006;6:45.

Delacourt C et al. Computed tomography with normal chest radiograph in tuberculous infection. *Arch Dis Child* 1993;69(4):430–432.

De Villiers RVP, Andronikou S, Van de Westhuizen S. Specificity and sensitivity of chest radiographs in the diagnosis of paediatric pulmonary tuberculosis and the value of additional high-kilovolt radiographs. *Austral Radiol* 2004;48(2):148–153.

Farinha NJ et al. Tuberculosis of the central nervous system in children: A 20-year survey. *J Infect* 2000;41(1):61–68.

Girgis NI et al. Tuberculosis meningitis, Abbassia Fever Hospital-Naval Medical Research Unit No. 3-Cairo, Egypt, from 1976 to 1996. *Am J Trop Med Hyg* 1998;58(1):28–34.

Graham SM, Daley HM, Ngwira B. Finger clubbing and HIV infection in Malawian children. *Lancet* 1997;349(9044):31.

Ling DI et al. Incremental value of T-SPOT.TB for diagnosis of active pulmonary tuberculosis in children in a high-burden setting: A multivariable analysis. *Thorax* 2013;68(9):860–866.

Madhi SA et al. Increased disease burden and antibiotic resistance of bacteria causing severe community-acquired lower respiratory tract infections in human immunodeficiency virus type 1-infected children. *Clin Infect Dis* 2000;31(1):170–176.

Mandalakas AM et al. Interferon-gamma release assays and childhood tuberculosis: Systematic review and meta-analysis. *Int J Tuberc Lung Dis* 2011;15(8):1018–1032.

Marais BJ et al. Diversity of disease in childhood pulmonary tuberculosis. *Ann Trop Paediatr* 2005;25(2):79–86.

Marais BJ et al. TB contact screening: Which way to go? [Correspondence]. *Int J Tuberc Lung Dis* 2009;13(12):1576–1577.

Marais BJ et al. The burden of childhood tuberculosis: A public health perspective. *Int J Tuberc Lung Dis* 2005;9(12):1305–1313.

Marais BJ et al. The natural history of childhood intra-thoracic tuberculosis: A critical review of literature from the pre-chemotherapy era. *Int J Tuberc Lung Dis* 2004;8(4):392–402.

Marais BJ et al. Well defined symptoms are of value in the diagnosis of childhood pulmonary tuberculosis. *Arch Dis Child* 2005;90(11):1162–1165.

Marais BJ et al. The spectrum of disease in children treated for tuberculosis in a highly endemic area [Unresolved Issues]. *Int J Tuberc Lung Dis* 2006;10(7):732–738.

Martineau AR et al. A single dose of vitamin D enhances immunity to mycobacteria. *Am J Respir Crit Care Med* 2007;176(2):208–213.

National Institute for Health and Clinical Excellence, Tuberculosis: Clinical diagnosis and management of tuberculosis, and measures for its prevention and control. NICE clinical guideline 117, NICE, London, U.K., 2011. https://www.nice.org.uk/guidance/cg117/resources/guidance-tuberculosis-pdf. Accessed August 2015.

Nnoaham KE, Clarke A. Low serum vitamin D levels and tuberculosis: A systematic review and meta-analysis. *Int J Epidemiol* 2008;37(1):113–119.

Pickering L et al. *Red Book: 2012 Report of the Committee on Infectious Diseases.* American Academy of Pediatrics, Elk Grove Village, IL, 2012.

Reid JK et al. The effect of Neonatal Bacille Calmette–Guérin vaccination on purified protein derivative skin test results in Canadian Aboriginal Children. *CHEST J* 2007;131(6):1806–1810.

Schopfer K et al. The sensitivity of an interferon-gamma release assay in microbiologically confirmed pediatric tuberculosis. *Eur J Pediatr* 2014;173(3):331–336.

Sinclair D, Abba K, Grobler L, Sudarsanam TD. Nutritional supplements for people being treated for active tuberculosis. *Cochrane Database of Systematic Reviews* 2011, Issue 11. Art. No.: CD006086.

Smith KC. Tuberculosis in children. *Curr Probl Pediatr* 2001;31(1):5–30.

Thwaites G et al. British Infection Society guidelines for the diagnosis and treatment of tuberculosis of the central nervous system in adults and children. *J Infect* 2009;59(3):167–187.

Thwaites GE, Hien TT. Tuberculous meningitis: Many questions, too few answers. *Lancet Neurol* 2005;4(3):160–170.

Wang L et al. A meta-analysis of the effect of Bacille Calmette–Guérin vaccination on tuberculin skin test measurements. *Thorax* 2002; 57(9):804–809.

World Health Organization. *Rapid Advice. Treatment of Tuberculosis in Children*. WHO, Geneva, Switzerland, 2010.

Yaramiş A et al. Central nervous system tuberculosis in children: A review of 214 cases. *Pediatrics* 1998;102(5):e49.

Zar HJ et al. Induced sputum versus gastric lavage for microbiological confirmation of pulmonary tuberculosis in infants and young children: A prospective study. *Lancet* 2005;365(9454):130–134.

6

Treatment

RAHULDEB SARKAR

GENERAL PRINCIPLES OF TREATMENT

BRIEF HISTORY OF TB TREATMENT

1. From the days of patients dying without treatment, to the days of sanatorium and trying to cure them with rest, diet and fresh air, and then sometimes with surgery, to the big leap made in the 1940s with the invention of the first antitubercular agent and then standardising gradually the regimen of multiple drug therapy globally, human civilisation has seen major advances in tuberculosis (TB) management in the last century.

2. In the last two decades, a major drive has been seen by the World Health Organization to reduce the prevalence of TB worldwide through the implementation of *directly observed treatment* as part of the effort of achieving one of the major Millennium Development Goals.

3. New challenges have also been faced with emergences of multidrug-resistant TB (MDR-TB) and extensively drug-resistant TB (XDR-TB) and advances have also been made at the same time with invention of rapid diagnostic assays of TB strains with resistance potential.

CURRENT WORLD HEALTH ORGANIZATION GOALS OF TB TREATMENT

1. To cure the patient and restore the quality of life and productivity
2. To prevent death from active TB or its late effects
3. To prevent the relapse of TB
4. To reduce the transmission of TB to others
5. To prevent the development and transmission of drug resistance

DEFINITIONS OF TREATMENT

1. Having a clear idea about various definitions at the outset in the area of TB cases helps us understand the treatment recommendations in different groups of TB patients by promoting a universal terminology in the field.

2. Definitions depending on bacteriological result
   a. *Smear-positive pulmonary TB*: If one or more sputum samples at the beginning of treatment are positive for acid fast bacilli.
   b. *Smear-negative pulmonary TB*: If the patient has smear-negative but culture-positive sputum (at least two specimens). The definition applies to patients who have been put on full anti-TB treatment by a clinician and has radiological features consistent with active pulmonary TB.

3. Definitions based on previously received treatment
   a. *New cases*: These are the patients with no prior history of TB treatment or are the patients who had TB treatment for less than 1 month.
   b. *Previously treated cases*
      Relapse: These patients had their treatment completed and were initially cured.
      Treatment failure: When treatment is completed but the patient has failed to become culture negative.
      Default: These patients dropped out of treatment after at least 1 month of their treatment.

4. Definitions based on microbial drug resistance
   a. *Drug resistant TB*: TB cases resistant to any number of antitubercular drugs
   b. *MDR-TB*: TB isolates resistant to at least isoniazid and rifampicin
   c. *XDR-TB*: Isolates resistant to isoniazid, rifampicin, as well as fluoroquinolone and either aminoglycosides or capreomycin
   d. Isolates that are resistant to all locally tested drugs have been termed as *totally drug-resistant* TB. The limitation of definition is that the studies describing these isolates did not include susceptibility to all the second-line agents, and often the drug susceptibility testing (DST) to all the second-line agents is not reliable. The WHO does not currently endorse this term.

5. The aim of treatment is to achieve both bactericidal activity in the first few weeks (i.e. rapidly reducing bacterial burden) and then to achieve sterilisation (i.e. eliminating persistent organisms) in later weeks. A combination of drugs is needed to achieve clinical cure as natural populations of bacteria in a diseased host are suspected to have wide heterogeneity in their characteristics (Figures 6.1 and 6.2).

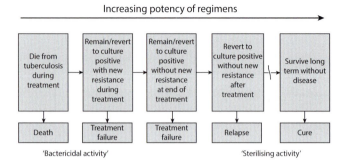

Figure 6.1 Hierarchy of clinical outcomes of tuberculosis treatment. As treatment regimens improve in their performance, preventing mortality and resistance by reducing bacillary burden within the first few weeks ('bactericidal activity') becomes less critical while eliminating persisting organisms during the remaining months of treatment ('sterilising activity') becomes crucial to long-term success.

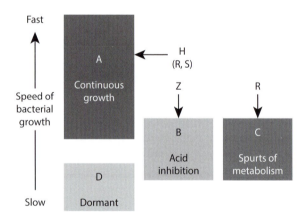

Figure 6.2 The subpopulations hypothesis of tuberculosis treatment. Natural populations of mycobacteria in a diseased host with a high bacillary burden are believed to be heterogeneous in their physiological characteristics and microenvironment. Consequently, drugs with a range of physico-chemical properties and mechanisms of action are needed to ensure complete elimination of all subpopulations and clinical treatment success. (From Canetti G, *Tubercle*, 43, 301, 1962; Mitchison DA, *Chest*, 76(6 Suppl), 771, 1979.)

PHARMACOLOGY OF FIRST-LINE DRUGS

1. Table 6.1 outlines the usual dose range, mechanism of actions, contra-indications and side effects of the first- and second-line antitubercular medications.
2. Abbreviations used in the following text: isoniazid, H; rifampicin, R; pyrazinamide, Z; ethambutol, E; streptomycin, S.
3. The first-line drugs should be taken 30 minutes before meals, but anorexia, nausea and abdominal pain can be caused by H, R or Z, and hence taking these drugs with small meals or just before bedtime may be helpful.

DRUG SUSCEPTIBILITY TESTING

CONVENTIONAL DRUG SUSCEPTIBILITY TESTING (DST)

1. This involves the traditional culture-based growth of the organism in drug-free and drug-containing media.
2. This method is time consuming and can take up nearly from 3 weeks to 2 months.
3. However, it is still regarded as the gold standard but is losing its role in detecting drug resistance in a short time to the rapid diagnostic assays.

RAPID DRUG SUSCEPTIBILITY TESTING

1. This method involves detecting certain nucleic acid sequences in the mycobacterial genome. In addition to being able to differentiate *Mycobacterium tuberculosis* (MTB) from other environmental mycobacteria, it can also detect mutation associated with drug resistance.
2. *GeneXpert MTB/RIF*: This is a nucleic acid amplification technique which is able to detect the *rpoB* gene of *MTB*. This method can correctly identify up to 98% of smear-positive cases, 72% of smear-negative but culture-positive cases and 98% of rifampicin resistance.
3. *MTBDRplus*: This assay is capable of detecting INH (*katG* and *inhA* genes) and rifampicin resistance (*rpoB* gene).
4. These test results should be interpreted with caution in a low prevalence area for MDR, as there is a potential for false positives.

Table 6.1 First- and second-line antitubercular drugs

Drug	Daily dose in mg/kg (max/day)	3/week dose in mg/kg	Mechanism of action	Toxicity
Isoniazid (oral/IM/IV)[a]	5 (300)	10 (900)	Bactericidal, rapidly absorbed, t½ in 1–3 hours	Skin rash, active/unstable liver disease/jaundice, peripheral neuropathy, drowsiness
Rifampicin (oral/ IV)[b]	10 (600)	10 (600)	Bactericidal (intra-/extracellular); inhibits DNA-dependent RNA polymerase; mammalian RNA polymerase does not bind rifampicin	Skin rash, jaundice, and AKI; reduces serum levels of many drugs including antiepileptics and oral contraceptives
Pyrazinamide[c]	25	35	Nicotinamide analogue, weakly bactericidal, strong sterilising activity in inflammatory tissue	Skin rash, jaundice, hyperuricemia and exacerbation of gout
Ethambutol[d]	15	30	Synthetic, bacteriostatic	Visual impairment, impairment of colour vision

(Continued)

Table 6.1 (Continued) First- and second-line antitubercular drugs

Drug	Daily dose in mg/kg (max/day)	3/week dose in mg/kg	Mechanism of action	Toxicity
Streptomycin (IM, can be given IV)[e]	15 (body weight <50 kg–500 mg)	15 (1000)	First antitubercular agent to be invented; derived from *Streptomyces griseus* and is bactericidal	Skin rash, deafness, dizziness, increased ototoxicity and nephrotoxicity in renal insufficiency

Notes:

[a] Pyridoxine should be given to the at-*risk* group; clinical and LFT monitoring in people with liver disease should be done; this raises serum levels of antiepileptics, e.g. phenytoin and carbamazepine, and hence their serum level. It can be used in pregnancy.

[b] Flu syndrome can be caused by intermittent rifampicin dosing; regularising the drug usually is helpful. This should be taken 30 minutes before meals. Resistance develops rapidly unless used with other antimicrobials. This causes orange staining of body secretions.

[c] Glycaemic control may become unstable; can be used in pregnancy; to be used in three/week regimen in renal failure patients; and does not work against *M. bovis*.

[d] In creatinine clearance <30 mL/min; to be used in three/week regimen.

[e] Must be used by deep IM injection, but cannot be used in pregnancy and myasthenia gravis. Ideal trough level, when it can be measured, is to be less than 4 mcg/mL; protective gloves help prevent sensitisation dermatitis.

TREATMENT OF PULMONARY TB

GENERAL ASPECTS

1. It is vital that a suitable sample is obtained for microbiological testing before initiating the treatment to establish the diagnosis as well as to establish any drug resistance of the isolate.
2. However, it must be recognised that despite the best efforts of the clinician, it may not be possible to obtain suitable microbiological samples and confirm the disease by a culture-positive result, and sometimes it is necessary to treat TB empirically with a pragmatic approach if the clinical and radiological picture fits with the disease in appropriate epidemiological setting.
3. The importance of good nutrition should be emphasised in the treatment of TB; in addition to the current drug regimen, a balanced nutritional intake is an integral part of TB management.

NEW CASES

INITIAL DIAGNOSIS

1. Ideally DST should be performed in all cases before treatment.
2. If resource does not allow doing DST in all cases, all new case *should* have DST in a country where prevalence of MDR in new cases is >3%.
3. If DST is not possible at all, two sputa for microscopy ± CXR (relevant in most settings) are recommended.

DRUG REGIMEN

1. 2HRZE/4HR (2 months of intensive and 4 months of continuation treatment).
2. Pyridoxine should be added at a dose of 20 mg/day in diabetic and cirrhotics patients, patients with renal failure or other malnourished patients and pregnant patients.
3. In a high isoniazid-resistance setting, the regimen should be 2HRZE/4HRE.
4. One notable exception is if the patient has acquired the disease from a MDR patient, then the treatment should be with empirical MDR regimen or as per DST result of the index case. Sputum for DST should be sent from the new case.

DOSING FREQUENCY

1. The best dosing frequency is daily. However, this is often not possible due to practical reasons.
2. The next best option is a daily intensive phase followed by three times a week intensive phase.
3. In extreme circumstances, if daily treatment is not feasible at all, three times a week regimen may be acceptable only if all the dosage is directly observed and the patient is not HIV positive and is not in a HIV prevalent area.

MONITORING DURING/AFTER TREATMENT

1. Patients should have their body weight monitored.
2. If sputum smear at the end of 2 months (even if the initial sputum smear was negative) is positive, repeat smear at the end of 3 months, and if positive still, send for culture and DST.
3. Repeat sputum smear at the end of 5 months.

SPECIAL SITUATIONS

1. In a setting with high isoniazid resistance, the regimen should be 2HRZ/4HRE.
2. CNS, joint or bone disease should be treated with longer regimen (see 'Treatment of Extrapulmonary TB' section).
3. Pyridoxine should be given at a dosage of 10 mg to HIV, diabetic, alcoholic and malnourished patients and to patients with liver disease and chronic kidney disease.

TREATMENT FAILURES

1. In a patient who is culture positive after 3 months of treatment of standard therapy, drug resistance should be suspected and treatment regimen changed accordingly.

Relapsed cases

BACKGROUND TO RELAPSED CASES

1. When there is a high suspicion of MDR-TB, the next management plans depend upon the known information on the HIV prevalence in the country. However, patients relapsing/ defaulting after their second course of treatment are already at high risk of MDR.

2. There is a 50%–94% chance of MDR, if someone has failed a 6-month regimen containing rifampicin.
3. *Initial diagnosis*: The diagnostic specimen (usually sputum) should be sent for DST and treatment should be started while waiting for the result of the DST. If available, rapid molecular DSTs are preferable (to enable the clinician to get the results within days).

DRUG REGIMEN

1. In a low MDR prevalence setting, 2HRZES/1HRZE/5HRE regimen can be used in patients relapsing after their first course of treatment.
2. All other patients should be started on empirical MDR regimen (see 'Multidrug-Resistant TB' section) and then the treatment can be modified as and when DST results arrive.

DOSING FREQUENCY

1. This should ideally be daily.
2. In other cases, intensive phase should be given daily with thrice a week continuation phase. Thrice a week intensive case should only be practised in patients who can be directly observed by the personnel.

MONITORING DURING/AFTER TREATMENT

1. For the retreatment regimen (2HRZES/1HRZE/5HRE), sputum smear should be done at the end of the intensive phase (after 3 months), and if positive, DST should be done.
2. If the sputum is negative at 3 months, then sputum smear should be done after 5 months (from initiation), and if positive, DST should be done.
3. If the 5-month sputum is negative, sputum smear is to be repeated after the completion of the treatment (8 months).
4. Smear positivity at 5 months or later, or finding of MDR at any point through DST, is defined as treatment failure.

HIV CO-INFECTION

BACKGROUND TO TREATMENT

1. Case fatality rate and drug resistance are higher among HIV-positive patients with TB and it is important that robust TB diagnostic procedure

is in place for people living with HIV. Active case finding helps identify TB at an earlier stage.

2. TB is also an AIDS-defining illness and anti-retroviral therapy (ART) should be started as soon as possible if TB is diagnosed in a HIV-positive patient.

3. There can be two potential situations with regard to HIV status. The patient in whom TB is being considered can either be known HIV positive or he or she might be living in a HIV prevalent setting and, therefore, a HIV suspect.

4. HIV testing and counselling should be offered to all patients with TB, especially in high prevalence settings and in *at-risk individuals* (*provider initiated* with opt-out option by patient if they did not want to be tested). This should be extended to household members as well. Furthermore, HIV prevention information should be provided to all TB patients.

INITIAL DIAGNOSIS (BOTH IN KNOWN HIV-POSITIVE AND HIV SUSPECTS)

1. HIV-positive patients can lack typical clinical or radiological pictures of TB and they have higher chance of having sputum negative and extra-pulmonary TB.

2. Performing chest x-ray in initial sputum smear–negative HIV-positive patients has an important role.

3. Performing DST at the start of TB treatment for HIV-positive patients is important. If this is not possible with available resources, at least this should be provided to previously treated patients.

4. HIV-positive contacts of known TB patients should be screened for TB. If screening is negative, they should be offered isoniazid prophylaxis.

5. Similarly, provider-initiated screening should be offered to household contacts and to TB patients with HIV.

DRUG REGIMEN

1. The regimen is similar to the regimen described in the previous section for new patients.

2. At least 6 months of therapy is needed. There are, however, some weak data supporting the treatment duration of 8 months.

3. Once on TB therapy, cotrimoxazole prophylaxis for *Pneumocystis jiroveci* is to be given to all TB patients with HIV irrespective of CD4 count.
4. Cotrimoxazole should be followed by initiation of ART within 8 weeks of initiation of antitubercular treatment. This should be done irrespective of CD4 count.
5. Immune reconstitution syndrome after initiation of ART is an important phenomenon to be aware of. This is due to rebuilding of the patient's immune system and can present with pyrexia, increased pulmonary infiltrate, lymphadenopathy, worsening of pre-existing inflammation and should resolve with a conservative management without the clinician having to stop ART. However, other differentials should be excluded. These include other opportunistic infection and TB treatment failure.

DOSING FREQUENCY

1. Three times a week intensive phase is not an option in HIV positives or suspects (increased chance of relapse) and they should receive the treatment daily.
2. Daily treatment is best in the continuation phase as well; however, if not possible, three times a week treatment can be given with strict direct supervision.

MONITORING DURING/AFTER TREATMENT

1. Monitoring is same as in non-HIV patients.
2. One needs to be aware of the interactions between antitubercular (mainly rifampicin) and ARTs. These drugs and cotrimoxazole often share the same side effects.

FURTHER CONSIDERATIONS IN HIV CO-INFECTION

1. In this group, a diagnosis of TB should alert the physician of the possibility of ART failure.
2. Consider modifying ARTs for drug–drug interactions with antitubercular agents.
3. In the non-nucleoside reverse transcriptase inhibitors, efavirenz should be chosen over nevirapine as the concentration of the later can be reduced by rifampicin.

TREATMENT OF EXTRAPULMONARY TB

1. Globally 10%–20% of all TB cases suffer from extrapulmonary disease according to the global TB report by WHO in 2012. Importantly, this can be associated with positive HIV status.
2. All extrapulmonary TB patients should have testing for HIV co-infection.
3. All patients should also have sputum smear (where possible) and chest radiograph as extrapulmonary TB can be associated with pulmonary disease. Along with diagnosing pulmonary TB, this can also guide the clinician in deciding the patient's infective potential.
4. Table 6.2 summarises salient points in the management of extrapulmonary TB according to WHO guidance.

MANAGING ADVERSE EFFECTS OF TREATMENT

MANAGING SYSTEMIC ADVERSE EFFECTS OF TB TREATMENT

1. Minor systemic symptoms should not make the clinician stop treatment. These can be in the form of itching, in which case antihistamine agents can be tried. Otherwise, the patient can develop mild nausea, anorexia, nausea and abdominal pain (in absence of jaundice), and taking the drugs with small meals or at bedtime usually helps in resolving the symptoms.
2. Mild drowsiness may be associated with isoniazid and again administration of the drug at bedtime helps in this situation.
3. Development of rash, however, should prompt the clinician to stop anti-TB medication and then to reintroduce the drugs one at a time and monitor response.
4. Rifampicin causes orange discolouration of bodily secretions, including urine, and patients should be counselled about this pretreatment to avoid undue panic. A flu-like illness can be associated with intermittent dosing of rifampicin and taking the drug daily usually should be enough to resolve this.
5. Three Ds (dizziness, deafness and decreasing urine output) can be associated with streptomycin and should prompt the clinician to stop the drug.

Table 6.2 Treatment of extrapulmonary tuberculosis

Site	Diagnostic specimen	Duration	Regimen
Tubercular meningitis[a]	CSF (other than cultures, molecular probe assays have sensitivity of nearly 60% and specificity of >95%)	12 months (for drug-sensitive isolate, 18–24 months is needed for drug-resistant TB)	2 HRSZ/10HR; 12 mg dexamethasone for 3 weeks initially, then tapered over next 3 weeks
Tubercular pericarditis[b]	Echocardiogram, calcification of pericardium in CXR, pericardial fluid	6 months	2HRZE/4HR; 1 mg/kg prednisolone for a month, gradually tapered over next 2 months
Tubercular peritonitis	Ascitic fluid microbiology, lymphocytic peritoneal fluid, laparoscopy/peritoneal biopsy, adenosine deaminase in peritoneal fluid, imaging lymph nodes. Resolution of the sinus can be achieved by antitubercular therapy alone.	6 months	2HRZE/4HR

(Continued)

Table 6.2 (Continued) Treatment of extrapulmonary tuberculosis

Site	Diagnostic specimen	Duration	Regimen
Pleural TB[c]	Pleural fluid cytology/culture (usually lymphocyte > 50%); blind/thoracoscopic pleural biopsy	6 months	2HRZE/4HR (role of corticosteroid is not very clear); fluid drainage may be needed to resolve breathlessness; otherwise, the fluid usually gets absorbed spontaneously
Skeletal TB	Imaging, appropriate joint fluid culture, culture of material obtained from a draining sinus	6 months (if rifampicin cannot be used, 12 months regimen is needed)	2HRZE/4HR; surgery is an integral part of management in spinal disease or chest wall cold abscess to prevent neurological sequelae (Continued)

Table 6.2 (Continued) Treatment of extrapulmonary tuberculosis

Site	Diagnostic specimen	Duration	Regimen
Tubercular lymphadenitis[d] (nearly half the cause of lymphadenopathy in the developing world)	Microbiology of FNA of lymph node. If it is negative/normal, excision biopsy to increase diagnostic yield (unless the patient is HIV positive and has suspected disseminated TB or, infrastructurally, excision will take >2 weeks), the node to be sent to laboratory in normal saline	6 months	2HRZE/4HR
Genitourinary TB (painless haematuria or testicular swelling can often be the presenting complaint in a TB prevalent setting)	Urine culture for TB[e], imaging (e.g. intravenous pyelogram)	6 months	2HRZE/4HR

Notes:
a Consider surgical ventricular decompression for obstructive hydrocephalus.
b Pericardiocentesis is often required in addition to drug therapy. Pericardiectomy is needed for constrictive pericarditis with haemodynamic effects or at an early stage with patients with pericardial calcification.
c Often pleural effusion associated with TB can be due to a delayed hypersensitivity reaction. Therefore, in more than half of the cases, pleural fluid culture can be negative. Predominant cell type can also vary depending upon the timing of pleural aspiration in relation to disease onset (early aspiration can show a neutrophil predominant fluid). A pleural biopsy often increases the yield in culture.
d Treatment can be initiated on the basis of clinical suspicion, high prevalence of TB in the setting and a lymphocytic fluid. Sinus formation is frequent in TB lymphadenitis and FNA can be helpful in preventing this in large fluctuant.
e Sterile pyuria in routine culture should raise suspicion of renal TB.

MANAGING HEPATIC SIDE EFFECTS OF TB TREATMENT

1. Most first line antitubercular drugs or ATDs (H, R, Z) are potentially hepatotoxic and this can be a problem at any time during the treatment, but mainly in the intensive phase. This can be in the form of acute hepatitis, cholestasis or granulomatous hepatitis.

2. Individuals developing hepatotoxicity from TB treatment can have a range of symptoms from being asymptomatic to having abdominal pain, jaundice, nausea, vomiting or itching. Increasing age, female sex and racial difference can play a role in determining susceptibility to hepatotoxicity.

3. Preferably, a liver function test (LFT) should be done at the beginning of treatment, if the infrastructure permits. LFT should be repeated if symptoms suggestive of hepatic adverse effects develop. In case the alanine transaminase (ALT) rises above three times the baseline (or if the symptoms are severe), ATDs needs to be stopped.

4. ATDs should also be stopped if the ALT has gone up by more than five times the baseline without any symptom. After LFT comes back to the baseline, one drug at a time should be reinitiated.

5. If, however, the patient is so sick that it is not affordable to stop TB treatment, a complete non-hepatotoxic regimen should be initiated immediately after stopping usual TB therapy.

6. Rifampicin needs to be started first at a smaller dose, which needs to be built up to normal dose over the next 3–4 days. If the LFTs remain stable, then isoniazid should be added.

7. If LFTs remain stable after reinitiating H and R, it is probably wise to leave pyrazinamide from the regimen as that is likely to be the culprit drug in this scenario. Similarly, if the LFTs become abnormal at any stage after initiation of either H or R, the drug that preceded LFT abnormality should be omitted from the regimen. Some likely regimens are given in case the patient cannot tolerate any particular drug or a drug combination:

   a. Hepatotoxic response to R – 2HES/10HE
   b. Hepatotoxic response to H – 6–9RZE
   c. Hepatotoxic response to Z – 2HRE/7HR
   d. Hepatotoxic response to H and R – 18–24 SEF (fluoro)

MONITORING IN RESOURCE POOR SETTINGS

In settings with poor resources (where serial biochemical monitoring can be challenging) the following should be considered:

1. If LFT cannot be done at all, then one needs to wait for 2 weeks after jaundice and upper abdominal pain is settled before reinitiating ART.
2. If hepatic side effects develop in the intensive phase of quadruple therapy, pyrazinamide can be replaced with streptomycin.
3. If adverse effects develop during continuation phase, both H and R can be restarted after jaundice and upper abdominal pain have resolved to ensure completion of 4 months of continuation phase of HR.

PATIENTS WITH PRE-EXISTING LIVER DISEASE

1. Patients with history of viral hepatitis or viral carriage or alcoholics can be treated with usual drug regimens. However, they are at increased risk of developing hepatotoxicity and a baseline LFT is helpful.
2. In case of severe liver disease, baseline LFT should be done and if ALT is >3 times normal, then the regimens mentioned earlier in case of hepatotoxicity (with 2, 1 or no hepatotoxic agent in the regimen) should be used.

TREATING TB IN SPECIAL SITUATIONS

MANAGING TB IN PATIENTS WITH RENAL DYSFUNCTION

1. The quadruple regimen should remain the same in severe renal insufficiency.
2. In the three times a week regimen, the dose of ethambutol and pyrazinamide should be reduced to the dose of daily regimen (15 and 25 mg/kg, respectively) due to significant renal excretion of their metabolites.
3. Pyridoxine should to be used with a regimen containing isoniazid.
4. Streptomycin should be avoided, if possible.

MANAGING TB IN PREGNANCY AND IN LACTATING WOMEN

1. Pregnant women should be given the standard regimen of quadruple therapy.
2. Streptomycin should not be given in pregnancy, and the same is true for aminoglycosides.
3. Lactating women should also receive standard treatment while the baby should continue to breastfeed.
4. TB in the baby should be ruled out and then he or she should be given 6 months of isoniazid prophylaxis followed by BCG vaccination.

BCG INFECTION

BACKGROUND TO BCG INFECTION

1. BCG infection is an interesting phenomenon usually complicating the clinical picture following intravesical administration of BCG for the treatment of bladder cancer. This is manifested by high-grade pyrexia, pneumonitis or hepatic symptoms.
2. It can also cause localised inflammation anywhere in the genitourinary tract. Distal sites like vertebral bodies and bone marrow can also be affected. Sepsis can occur.
3. Non-caseating granuloma can be found in tissue specimens and findings of acid-fast bacilli (AFB) have also been documented. This is thought to be either due to hypersensitivity reaction or infective process. Diagnosis is made by tissue specimen staining or rarely by culture of *Mycobacterium bovis*. Radiology can show nodular pattern in the lungs. High index of clinical suspicion is needed.

TREATMENT OF BCG INFECTION

1. Treatment is with symptomatic management in mild form of disease, in the early phase immediately after BCG instillation. If there are systemic symptoms of TB (fever, night sweat), ART, usually with corticosteroids, needs to be initiated.

2. Pyrazinamide does not act against *M. bovis* and, therefore, should not be used. For localised disease (cystitis), monotherapy with isoniazid for 2–3 weeks should be given. If the patient does not respond in the initial few days, a combination therapy with H and R for 3 months is needed.
3. For disseminated infection, 3–6 months of combination therapy is needed. In the initial phase of treatment, glucocorticoid can be used with caution.

SURGICAL TREATMENT

1. There used to be widespread role of surgical treatment in TB in the early part of twentieth century prior to development of antitubercular chemo-therapeutic agents. This included therapeutic pneumothorax, phrenic nerve crush, plombage or thoracoplasty and they played a major role in treating this potentially fatal condition at that time (Figures 6.3 and 6.4).
2. In the current day practice, the role of surgery is limited in the following areas:
   a. Treating complication of pre-existing TB (haemoptysis, bronchiec-tatic lobe)
   b. Diagnostic process (e.g. lymph node excision, tissue biopsy)
   c. Spinal stabilisation in spinal TB
   d. Relieving of hydrocephalus in TB meningitis through shunts
   e. Treatment of MDR-TB (i.e. pneumonectomy or lobectomy should be considered in MDR-TB or XDR-TB that does not respond to drug therapy) (Figures 6.5 through 6.7).

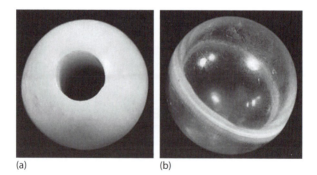

(a)   (b)

Figure 6.3 Plombage was previously undertaken to facilitate 'collapse therapy', using materials such as 'polystan balls' (a) and 'lucite balls' (b).

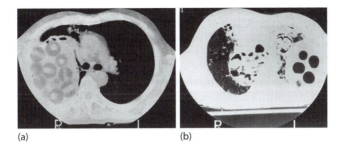

(a)   (b)

Figure 6.4 Computed tomographic cuts showing the characteristic appearances of (a) 'polystan balls' and (b) 'lucite balls'. In addition, this patient also had extensive cavitation and fungal colonisation.

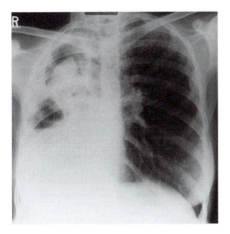

Figure 6.5 The chest x-ray of a patient with total destruction of the right lung following tuberculosis. The largest cavity has been colonised by a large fungal ball. Repeated haemoptysis required pleuropneumonectomy.

TREATMENT OF DRUG-RESISTANT TB

1. Resistance to chemotherapeutic agents is a problem similar to other antibiotic resistances in various other microorganisms and is a major public health hazard of the twenty-first century. A basic understanding of the second-line antitubercular agents is important to be able to design a regimen for MDR-TB or XDR-TB.

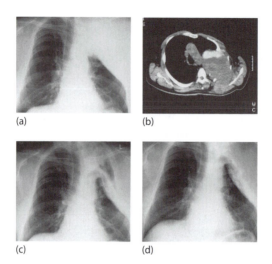

Figure 6.6 (a) The chest x-ray of a patient presenting with chest wall pain and a mass 40 years after plombage for tuberculosis. A sarcoma was suspected, but (b) the computed tomography scan shows the underlying plombage expanding through the chest wall. (c) After the evacuation of the shredded plastic plombage material, drainage shows the size of the residual cavity. (d) Six months later, the patient accepted surgery to obliterate the space by trimming thoracoplasty and omental transfer, with complete resolution.

2. Basic information on second-line drugs is detailed in Table 6.3.
3. Some examples of regimens for mono-resistance are as follows:
   a. Isoniazid resistance – 2HRZE/4HRE or 2RZ/7RE
   b. Rifampicin resistance – 9HSZ or 12HZE
   c. Pyrazinamide resistance – 9HR
   d. Ethambutol resistance – 2HRZ/4HR

MULTIDRUG-RESISTANT TB

SUSPICION AND ESTABLISHMENT OF MDR CASES

1. MDR should be suspected based on previous treatment failure, resistance profile of the index case or local epidemiological data (high incidence of resistance) including patient's HIV status.

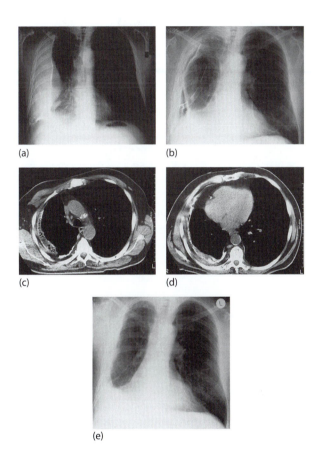

Figure 6.7 (a) The chest x-ray of a patient with right chest pain many years after 'collapse therapy' for tuberculosis. The presence of the wound and the extensive pleural calcification should have alerted the physician to the underlying cause. The patient neglected to mention the history, and malignancy was suspected. (b) Eventually, rather inadequate drainage was performed by a surgeon who attempted pleurodesis. (c, d) The computed tomographic cuts, clearly show the residual space and heavily calcified visceral and parietal cortex. The patient was reluctant to accept surgery and persisted with drainage for 1 year. (e) The chest x-ray after corrective surgery shows the space obliterated by decortication, omental transfer and a myoplastic flap to the apex of the space.

Table 6.3 Treatment of drug-resistant tuberculosis

Group 1 drugs	
Pyrazinamide	• Most potent and best tolerated.
Ethambutol	• If a drug was present in a previous
Rifabutin	regimen that failed, its efficacy in that
	patient should be questioned despite
	favourable DST.
	• Rifabutin has cross resistance with
	rifampicin.
Group 2 drugs (injectables)	
Kanamycin (Km)	• Km and Am are the first choice (they
Amikacin (Am)	have high rate of cross resistance).
Capreomycin	• Km is cheap.
	• If an isolate is resistant to kanamycin, or if
	DRS data show high rates of resistance
	to amikacin and kanamycin, capreomycin
	(a polypeptide) should be used.
	• Capreomycin can cause significant
	hypokalaemia and therefore needs close
	monitoring.
Group 3 drugs (fluoroquinolones)	
Levofloxacin	• All patients should have a group 3 drug
Moxifloxacin	(if the isolate is susceptible or if the
Gatifloxacin	agent is thought to have efficacy).
	• Levo or Moxi are the agents of choice.
	• Cipro is no longer recommended.
Group 4 drugs (oral bacteriostatic second-line agents)	
Ethionamide	• Bacteriostatic.
Prothionamide	• Ethionamide is added first because of its
PAS	low cost.
Cycloserine	• Ethionamide has little effect in patients
Terizidone	treated previously for MDR-TB.
Thioacetazone	• If cost is no bar, PAS can be added
(Ethionamide can cause	instead of ethionamide (better tolerated
hepatotoxicity,	as enteric-coated preparation).
neurotoxicity and	
hypothyroidism.)	

(Continued)

Table 6.3 (*Continued*) Treatment of drug-resistant tuberculosis

Group 4 drugs (oral bacteriostatic second-line agents)	
(Cycloserine can cause adverse psychiatric effects.) (Thioacetazone can cause Steven–Johnson syndrome in HIV-positive population.)	• Combination of ethionamide and PAS causes hypothyroidism and gastrointestinal side effect and hence only combined if three group four agents are needed (ethionamide, cycloserine and PAS). • Terizidone can be used instead of cycloserine, if it causes psychiatric side effects.
Group 5 drugs (agents with unclear role in the treatment of drug-resistant TB)	
Clofazimine (Cfz), linezolid (Lzd), co-amoxiclav, thioacetazone (thz), imipenem, cilastatin, high-dose INH, clarithromycin	• Not recommended by WHO for routine use • Can be used in cases where it is impossible to design a regimen from groups 1 to 4 (e.g. XDR-TB) • Should be used in consultation with an expert

2. WHO update in 2011 on management of drug-resistant TB recommends rapid DST testing for all patients, subject to available resources, to facilitate early recognition of MDR cases.
3. Rifampicin resistance on Xpert/MTB/RIF should prompt the clinician to consider MDR treatment, unless the setting has a low rifampicin resistance, in which case the result should be confirmed with phenotypic DST or line probe assay to avoid false-positive result.
4. If resources do not allow rapid DST on all patients, this is recommended strongly for high-risk groups for developing MDR-TB.
5. Reliability of susceptibility testing is not 100% in all drugs other than H, R, injectables and fluoroquinolones.
6. Even at an individual level, WHO suggests that the resistance pattern might vary and expand from the time the culture specimen was taken to the time the culture is reported because of the patient being on a suboptimal regimen during this time period.

CHOOSING/DESIGNING A REGIMEN AS PER CURRENT WHO GUIDANCE

1. Initial MDR regimen should be guided by the country-specific empirical MDR regimen (based on the local resistance profile) until conventional DST result comes back.
2. An individually tailored regimen can be initiated upon the availability of the result from conventional DST, which gives the clinician the knowledge about resistance to first- and second-line agents.
3. The regimen should contain at least four second-line drugs, along with pyrazinamide during the intensive phase.
4. In an area, empirical MDR regimen needs to be continuously updated depending on the available DST data on second-line agents.
5. More than four drugs can be started if the initial four drugs cannot be relied upon entirely to provide a good cover (in case of unknown susceptibility or if drugs had to be chosen keeping in mind interactions or patient comorbidity, which renders the chosen regimen less potent).
6. Drugs from various groups should be used while designing a regimen:
   a. Pyrazinamide should be used during intensive phase.
   b. There should be one injectable agent (kanamycin is cheap, otherwise amikacin).
   c. There should be a higher generation fluoroquinolone (not ciprofloxacin).
   d. Ethionamide should be a part of the regimen.
   e. Cycloserine should also be used, or otherwise PAS, if cycloserine cannot be used.

DURATION OF TREATMENT

1. The total duration is usually >20 months.
2. Intensive phase comprises at least 6 months and at least 4 months after the patient had become sputum smear and culture negative (intensive phase is defined as the duration through which injectable agent should be used).
3. Similarly, WHO suggests continuing therapy for a minimum of 18 months of culture conversion (conversion is said to have occurred if two samples taken 30 days apart are both smear and culture negative).

MONITORING DURING MDR THERAPY

1. Close monitoring of the patient for response to treatment is required and is as follows:
2. Monthly sputum smear and culture testing should be done until culture conversion, starting after 2 months of initiation of therapy.
3. If the smear is positive at the end of third month, culture and DST should be done.
4. Following conversion, monthly sputum smear and culture test should be done every 3 months.
5. Parallel clinical assessment should also be carried out every month before conversion and quarterly after conversion.

SETTING OF TREATMENT

1. In the latest guidance in this topic in 2011, WHO recommended an ambulatory non-hospital-based treatment approach for this group of patients.
2. In a sicker group of patients, hospitalisation may be necessary.

TREATMENT OF XDR-TB

1. Treatment of XDR-TB management should only be initiated in specialist centres with significant experience in treatment.
2. Conventional DST is the gold standard in diagnosing XDR as the sensitivity for rapid assays for fluoroquinolones and injectables are low (e.g. all the mutations involved in drug resistance cannot yet be tested through his method).
3. Detailed history of previous anti-retroviral therapy (ART) drug use is very important.
4. Often around six agents are used.
5. Designing a regimen follows the same principle as designing MDR regimen.
6. The usual regimen should include any first-line agent the isolate is susceptible to, an injectable agent (depending on susceptibility) along with two to three second-line oral agents based on susceptibility.

7. One higher generation fluoroquinolone can be used despite resistance.
8. If sputum smear is positive despite several months of treatment, more than one agent should be added in.
9. Duration is 18 months after sputum conversion.
10. Monitoring is same as MDR-TB; CXR monitoring is also helpful.
11. There is a role for surgical resection of the affected areas in difficult cases; this has been shown to result in improved outcome, especially in localised disease.
12. ART must be started as soon as possible where appropriate.

NEW HORIZONS IN TB TREATMENT

1. The medical community is constantly thriving for newer weapons in the battle against TB, especially with emergence of new resistance patterns.
2. Furthermore, one of the major drawbacks in any TB regimen is the prolonged period that the patient has to take multiple medication with various potential side effects. This invariably raises issues around compliance and the lack of treatment adherence contributes, in turn, to drug resistance.
3. Therefore, it would be ideal to obtain newer agents which can inherently overcome the resistance of bacteria and also can be given in shorter courses.
4. The agents that are of promise and have been still shown to reduce early bactericidal activity are bedaquiline, delamanid and PA-824. They are being tested in combination with other first- and second-line agents to develop shorter courses.

LEARNING POINTS

1. Treatment of TB should ideally occur after microbiological confirmation and DST, but this may not always be possible.
2. The drug regimen chosen will depend on the site of infection, results of DST and local epidemiological data.
3. Surgical treatment of TB has a limited use in the modern setting.

4. Minor adverse effects should not lead to the termination of treatment but liver function should be monitored carefully.
5. MDR should be suspected based on previous treatment failure, resistance profile of the index case or local epidemiological data.
6. Drugs from different groups including the use of one injectable form should be considered when treating MDR-TB.
7. Management of MDR-TB should be initiated in specialist centres with significant experience in treatment.

FURTHER READING

Boehme CC et al. Rapid molecular detection of tuberculosis and rifampin resistance. *N Engl J Med* 2010;363:1005.

Davies PDO. *Clinical Tuberculosis*, 5th edn. CRC Press, Boca Raton, FL, 2014.

Dooley KE, Kim PS, Williams SD, Hafner R. TB and HIV therapeutics: Pharmacology research priorities. *AIDS Res Treat* 2012;2012:874083.

Johnson JL et al. Shortening treatment in adults with noncavitary tuberculosis and 2-month culture conversion. *Am J Respir Crit Care Med* 2009;180(6):558–563.

Johnston JC, Shahidi NC, Sadatsafavi M, Fitzgerald JM. Treatment outcomes of multidrug-resistant tuberculosis: A systematic review and meta-analysis. *PLoS One* 2009;4(9):e6914.

Lee M et al. Linezolid for treatment of chronic extensively drug-resistant tuberculosis. *N Engl J Med* 2012;367(16):1508–1518.

Lienhardt C et al. Efficacy and safety of a 4-drug fixed-dose combination regimen compared with separate drugs for treatment of pulmonary tuberculosis: The study C randomized controlled trial. *JAMA* 2011;305(14):1415–1423.

Mitchison DA. Basic mechanisms of chemotherapy. *Chest* 1979;76(6 Suppl): 771–781.

Peloquin CA. Therapeutic drug monitoring in the treatment of tuberculosis. *Drugs* 2002;62(15):2169–2183.

Shi W et al. Pyrazinamide inhibits trans-translation in *Mycobacterium tuberculosis*. *Science* 2011;333(6049):1630–1632.

Somoskovi A, Parsons LM, Salfinger M. The molecular basis of resistance to isoniazid, rifampin, and pyrazinamide in Mycobacterium tuberculosis. *Respir Res* 2001;2(3):164–168.

Tiemersma EW, Van der Werf MJ, Borgdorff MW, Williams BG, Nagelkerke NJD. Natural history of tuberculosis: Duration and fatality of untreated pulmonary tuberculosis in HIV negative patients: A systematic review. *PLoS One* 2011;6(4):e17601.

Vilchèze C et al. Transfer of a point mutation in Mycobacterium tuberculosis inhA resolves the target of isoniazid. *Nat Med* 2006;12(9):1027–1029.

Wittes R, Klotz L, Kosecka U. Severe bacillus Calmette–Guerin cystitis responds to systemic steroids when antituberculous drugs and local steroids fail. *J Urol* 1999;161:1568.

7

New drugs for TB

SYED MURTAZA H KAZMI

INTRODUCTION

1. Tuberculosis (TB) is a global pandemic and remains a persistent problem in the developing countries of Asia and Africa.
2. TB is one of the top three infectious disease killers worldwide. The WHO estimates that 2 billion people are infected with *Mycobacterium tuberculosis*, and at any given moment, more than 12 million people are suffering from an active infection.
3. The insufficient and inconsistent use of TB therapy has resulted in the emergence of multidrug-resistant TB (MDR-TB) in the last three decades. Once a TB strain is drug resistant, it can be

transmitted directly to others in the same manner as a drug-susceptible strain.

4. The more extreme variant of MDR-TB is extensively drug-resistant TB (XDR-TB), which was first recognized in 2006. According to WHO figures for the year 2010, 650,000 patients (out of 12 million prevalent TB patients) were estimated to be MDR-TB.

CURRENT TB TREATMENT

1. The current treatment of drug-susceptible TB consists of a 6-month regimen that includes isoniazid, rifampicin, pyrazinamide and ethambutol given daily for 2 months, followed by rifampicin and isoniazid for 4 months.

2. This standard regimen is based on a series of trials conducted by British Medical Research Council over 20 years that resulted in the permanent cure of more than 95% of trial participants.

3. This so-called short-course treatment has historically had a good success rate in treating TB.

4. In the real-world setting, however, the compliance and adherence to the treatment is a continual challenge faced by the health authorities worldwide. In addition, the full application of directly observed treatment short (DOTS) strategy is also becoming more difficult in resource-poor countries.

5. The current regimen includes drugs that are more than 40 years old; the last drug approved for TB was rifampicin that was discovered in 1963. Since then very few new classes of drugs have been evaluated as antituberculous agents.

6. The WHO declared TB a global emergency in 1993, which led to a revival of efforts to develop improved TB treatment.

7. The treatment of MDR-TB consists of second-line drugs, mostly in the form of injections that are given for 2 years or longer. The longer duration and a high toxicity profile lead to a poor compliance resulting in a poorer outcome.

8. The treatment options in XDR-TB are further limited due to resistance to most of the currently available drugs.

THE NEED FOR NEW DRUGS

Four main factors necessitate the development of new drugs for the treatment of TB.

INADEQUACY

1. The 6-months standard regimen requires a significant time to cure disease and has a significant side effect profile, both of which result in poor compliance.
2. The therapy is not currently adequate and has failed to halt disease spread globally.
3. The regimen is too complex to administer and puts an increasing burden on already resource limited public health authorities in the developing countries.
4. These factors combined lead to treatment failure, which are part of the reason why 1.4 million people die from TB annually.
5. A new shorter and simpler therapy regimen would help save millions of lives worldwide.
6. Current TB drugs have a number of interactions which need to be considered when they are being used (Table 7.1).

DRUG RESISTANCE

1. The last few decades have seen the continuous rise of MDR- and XDR-TB. These strains are the result of inadequate administration and interrupted treatment when patients stop taking medicine before the disease can be fully eradicated.
2. Today, direct transmission of the resistant strains is the most common way of MDR-TB and XDR-TB spread. A substantial increase in the notification of MDR-TB occurred since 2008.
3. The current treatment for these strains involves a more prolonged and complex regime of second-line drugs, mostly in the form of injectables. In addition, the use of these drugs is further limited by toxic side effects such as nephrotoxicity and ototoxicity with aminoglycosides, hepatotoxicity with ethionamide and dysglycaemia with gatifloxacin.

Table 7.1 Tuberculosis drug interactions

Drug X	Drug Y			
	Y increases X concentrations	Y decreases X concentrations	X increases Y concentrations	X decreases Y concentrations
Aminoglycosides[a]	None (except drug-induced renal failure)	None	None	None
Cycloserine	None (except drug-induced renal failure)	None	None	None
Ethambutol	None (except drug-induced renal failure)	Antacids	None	None
Ethionamide	None	None	(INH)	None
Fluoroquinolones[b]	None	Antacids Sucralphate Iron and other di- and trivalent cations	Theophylline (ciprofloxacin only)	None
Isoniazid	± Prednisolone	± Antacids	Carbamazepine Phenytoin ± Diazepam ± Warfarin	Enflurane
PAS	None	None	None	None
Pyrazinamide	None	Allopurinol	(Probenecid)	None

(Continued)

Table 7.1 (Continued) Tuberculosis drug interactions

Drug X	Drug Y			
	Y increases X concentrations	Y decreases X concentrations	X increases Y concentrations	X decreases Y concentrations
Rifamycins (most hepatically metabolized drugs can display lower concentrations when administered concurrently with rifamycins)[c]	Clarithromycin and rifabutin only: Fluconazole Itraconazole Voriconazole	Rifabutin only: Efavirenz Possibly nevirapine Possibly phenytoin	None	RIF ≥ RPNT> RBN Antidepressants β-Blockers Benzodiazepines Clarithromycin Calcium channel blockers Contraceptives (oral) Enalapril Fluvastatin Glucocorticoids Immunosuppressants Itraconazole Opiods Sulphonylureas Verapamil Voriconazole Warfarin

Note: See also references under individual drugs; INH, isoniazid; PAS, para-aminosalicylic acid; RBN, rifabutin; RIF, rifampicin; RPNT, rifapentine.

[a] Streptomycin, amikacin, kanamycin and the polypeptides capreomycin and viomycin.

[b] Ciprofloxacin, ofloxacin, levofloxacin, gatifloxacin and moxifloxacin.

[c] Rifampicin ≥ rifapentine (85% to >100%) > rifabutin (40%).

4. The cost of drug-resistant TB treatment is significant and poses a substantial challenge to health authorities and funding bodies. This demands a simpler and cheaper treatment regimen that can address emerging resistance.

HIV CO-INFECTION

1. HIV co-infection presents a serious challenge in the treatment of TB.
2. In high prevalence countries, the likelihood of HIV/AIDS patients contracting TB infection is increased significantly, thereby further increasing morbidity and mortality. TB co-infection can accelerate the progression of HIV infection.
3. HIV/TB co-infection complicates the selection of appropriate and effective treatment regime because (a) drug–drug interactions result in suboptimal levels of antiretrovirals (ARVs) and (b) toxic side effects raise safety concerns.
4. The main interaction between ARVs and TB therapy is the rifampicin-induced cytochrome P450 induction in the liver that results in increased metabolism and reduced therapeutic levels of many co-medications such as ARV protease inhibitors.
5. The increased pill burden for co-infected patients reduces compliance.
6. HIV patients with drug-resistant TB strains require treatment with second-line TB drugs, and to date there are no established studies that explore drug–drug interaction between ARVs and second-line anti-tuberculous medications.
7. The treatment options for dually infected patients are limited and complex. There is a clear need for developing newer drugs that act faster, avoid interaction with ARVs and are less toxic.

ECONOMIC BURDEN

1. Current treatment is struggling to control TB worldwide, which has a significant bearing on the global economy. It is estimated that world's poorest countries will lose $1–$3 trillion over the next 10 years due to TB.
2. The TB-endemic countries, where 94% of TB cases occur, are already overburdened and rely on donor countries to obtain TB drugs and treat their patients.

3. The burden of TB disease also slows down economic development with 75% of TB cases occurring during people's most productive years (15–54 years).
4. The economic drain on individual families is also very significant. The WHO calculates that the average TB patient loses 3–4 months of work time and up to 30% of yearly household earnings.
5. A shorter TB regimen would cut the expenses of TB care for over-stretched health-care systems. It may also reduce lost work time and minimize the economic impact of TB on individuals' lives.

DEVELOPING NEW DRUGS

CHALLENGES WITH DRUG DEVELOPMENT

1. In order to tackle TB pandemic effectively, faster-acting and affordable drugs are urgently needed.
2. Drugs are needed to better target the bacteria that survive (and are therefore not killed) within the first few weeks of bactericidal therapy which happens during current treatment.
3. The challenge of developing new drugs which can
   a. Shorten treatment duration (and therefore also increase compliance)
   b. Target MDR or XDR strains
   c. Simplify treatment by reducing the daily pill burden
   d. Lower dosing frequency (e.g. a once-weekly regimen)
   e. Be co-administered with HIV medications cause difficulties in drug discovery efforts
4. Earlier the situation remained the same due to lack of funding, but this has changed now as TB has been declared a global emergency.

ADVANCES IN DRUG DEVELOPMENT

1. The Working Group on New Drugs was formed in 2001 to facilitate global collaborations for the development of new TB drugs. The last decade, therefore, has seen encouraging advances in research and development in this area.
2. There are currently at least 10 compounds in clinical development: 6 in phase II and 4 in phase III trials.

In addition to individual drug testing, the first novel TB drug regimen also began clinical testing in 2010. This regimen, consisting of moxifloxacin, PA-824 and pyrazinamide, performed extremely well with mean 14-day early bactericidal activity comparable to the standard regimen, showing the potential for a single regimen to treat both drug-sensitive TB and MDR-TB in 4 months. This regimen is currently being tested in both TB and MDR-TB patients.

UPCOMING TB DRUGS

A number of drugs are being investigated for the treatment of TB. The following are some examples of drugs currently in phase II and III trials at the time of this writing.

RIFAPENTINE

1. Rifapentine is an attractive candidate for shortening TB therapy because it has a greater potency against *M. tuberculosis* and a longer half-life.
2. It is currently being tested comparing 12 once-weekly doses of rifapentine 900 mg + isoniazid 900 mg given by DOTS vs. 9 months of self-administered daily INH 300 mg in the treatment of latent TB in persons at high risk.
3. It is also being tested in phase II clinical trial for minimizing the drug-susceptible TB treatment to evaluate the antimicrobial activity and safety of an experimental intensive-phase (first 8 weeks of treatment) treatment regimen in which rifapentine is substituted for rifampin.

FLUOROQUINOLONES

1. Fluoroquinolones are used as second-line drugs in the treatment of MDR-TB. The newer agents in this class, *gatifloxacin* and *moxifloxacin*, have shown more potent activity against *M. tuberculosis* than the older compounds (ciprofloxacin and ofloxacin).
2. Moxifloxacin is currently being tested in phase III trial, namely REMoxTB. The trial is a randomized, double-blind, controlled study in which moxifloxacin is substituted for either ethambutol or isoniazid and is administered for a total of 4 months.

3. It aims to test whether a moxifloxacin-containing treatment regimen of just 4 months can cure drug-sensitive TB patients at rates that are non-inferior to those achieved with the standard 6-month TB regimen.
4. Gatifloxacin is also being tested in phase III trial that will evaluate the efficacy and safety of a gatifloxacin-containing regimen of 4 months duration for the treatment of pulmonary TB.

DELAMANID (OPC-67683)

1. Delamanid (OPC-67683), a nitro-dihydro-imidazooxazole derivative, is a new anti-TB medication that has shown potent activity against drug-resistant strains of *M. tuberculosis.*
2. A recently published study evaluated the efficacy of delamanid administered orally as 100 mg twice daily (BID) for 2 months followed by 200 mg once daily (QD) for 4 months in combination with an optimized background regimen (OBR) versus placebo with OBR during the 6-month intensive phase of MDR-TB treatment.
3. The results showed that delamanid was associated with an increase in sputum-culture conversion at 2 months among patients with MDR-TB. This finding suggests that delamanid could enhance treatment options for MDR-TB.
4. Phase III trial of safety and efficacy of delamanid for 6 months in patients with MDR-TB is currently enrolling.

BEDAQUILINE (TMC207)

1. TMC207 is a new agent being developed for TB treatment. It is a diarylquinoline investigational compound that offers a novel mechanism of anti-TB action by specifically inhibiting mycobacterial adenosine triphosphate synthase.
2. It has high *in vitro* activity against both drug-sensitive and drug-resistant MTB isolates and is also bactericidal against non-replicating tubercle bacilli. A phase II study in MDR patients is ongoing.

PA-824

1. PA-824 is also a new agent being developed for TB treatment. It is a nitroimidazole, a class of novel antibacterial agents.

2. Nonclinical studies have demonstrated important properties, particularly its novel mechanism of action and its activity against both drug-sensitive TB and MDR-TB. The development of PA-824 has progressed into phase II trial.

SUMMARY

1. The current regimen includes drugs that are more than 40 years old and the last major drug approved for TB treatment was rifampicin which was discovered in 1963.
2. Drug resistance, HIV co-infection and a lengthy complicated treatment regimen are some of the reasons why new drugs are needed.
3. There are at least 10 compounds in phase II or III clinical trials worldwide.

FURTHER READING

TB Alliance. A global partnership for TB drug development. www.tballiance.org. Accessed 25 July 2012.

Diacon, AH et al. 14-day bactericidal activity of PA-824, bedaquiline, pyrazinamide, and moxifloxacin combinations: A randomized trial. *The Lancet* 380(9846), 986–993.

Gler MT et al. Delamanid for multidrug-resistant pulmonary tuberculosis. *N Engl J Med* 2012 June 7;366(23):2151–2160.

Koul A et al. The challenge of new drug discovery for tuberculosis. *Nature* 2011 January 27;469(7331):483–490.

Lienhardt C et al. New drugs and new regimens for the treatment of tuberculosis: Review of the drug development pipeline and implications for national programmes. *Curr Opin Pulm Med* 2010 May;16(3):186–193.

Orenstein EW et al. Treatment outcomes among patients with multidrug-resistant tuberculosis: Systematic review and meta-analysis. *Lancet Infect Dis* 2009;9:153–161.

The Working Group on New Drugs (WGND). www.newtbdrugs.org. Accessed 25 July 2012.

Latent tuberculosis infection

MANISH GAUTAM

Case study 8.1

A 30-year-old male teaching assistant, KY, presented to the contact tracing clinic. His wife had been recently diagnosed with active pulmonary tuberculosis. He was asymptomatic; in particular there was no history of shortness of breath, cough, phlegm, hemoptysis, weight loss or reduced appetite. He was generally fit and well and had no significant medical history. He did not take any regular medication, was a non-smoker and consumed alcohol occasionally. On examination, there were no significant findings and his chest x-ray was normal. MY is the 70-year-old mother of KY. She also presented to the local contact tracing clinic as her son visited her on a regular basis. She was asymptomatic and well in herself, a non-smoker and retired chef. Her past medical history included hypertension, type 2 diabetes and pernicious anaemia. On examination there were no abnormal findings and her chest x-ray was normal. Do either KY or MY need screening for latent tuberculosis infection (LTBI)? If so, how would you screen them?

BACKGROUND TO LATENT TUBERCULOSIS INFECTION

1. The presence of quiescent mycobacteria in the absence of active infection, but with the potential to reactivate and cause disease, constitutes a diagnosis of latent tuberculosis infection (LTBI).

2. LTBI may represent tuberculosis disease that was previously present but not currently active, or tuberculosis infection, which has not progressed to cause disease.

3. For some who breathe in TB bacteria and become infected, the body is able to fight the bacteria and stop multiplication. In contrast to active TB infection, individuals with LTBI are asymptomatic.

4. Individuals with LTBI are not infectious and cannot spread the bacteria to others. However, if the mycobacteria become active in the body and begin to multiply, LTBI will progress to the disease and the individual will consequently present with typical symptoms.

5. In cases where a long period elapses between infection and development of disease, dormant bacilli are thought to remain in either the lung or other sites, which can 'reactivate' in favourable circumstances for the organism. Hence there remains a lifelong risk of progression to disease for all those with 'dormant' organisms.

6. The majority of exposed persons will kill off the inhaled bacteria. However, of those people presumed infected, there is a 10%–15% chance of developing clinical disease at some point in their lives.

7. The greatest chance of progressing to the disease is within the first 2 years after infection. The risk of developing clinical TB depends on both the risk of becoming infected and the risk of progressing to the disease after acquiring infection.

8. A number of risk factors have been identified as related to progression from LTBI to active TB:

a. Infection earlier in life may be associated with increased risks of progression and disease dissemination. About half of those who develop the clinical disease will do so within 5 years of the initial infection.

b. The presence of co-morbidity which reduces the host's immunological defence increases the risk of progression into active disease. For example, for HIV-infected patients, the chance of developing active TB within 5 years of infection is up to 50%.

c. Other risk factors include very old or very young patients, IV drug users, solid organ transplantation, malignancy, chronic renal failure or haemodialysis, gastrectomy, jejunoileal bypass, anti-TNF-alpha treatment, silicosis, diabetes, chemotherapy and immunosuppression.

DIAGNOSIS OF LTBI

WHO SHOULD BE TESTED FOR LTBI?

1. The rationale for testing LTBI lies in the identification of individuals who are at increased risk for the development of tuberculosis and, therefore, would benefit from treatment. In other words, testing for LTBI should be reserved for those in whom a positive result would prompt a decision to treat.

2. Individuals considered more likely to get TB disease include the following:

   a. Household and non-household close contacts (may include a boy-friend or girlfriend and frequent visitors to the home of the index case) of a person with TB disease

   b. Immunocompromised individuals

   c. New entrants from high incidence countries

   d. Contacts in an outbreak situation

   e. Healthcare workers

   f. Hard to reach groups (homeless shelters, prison or jails, or IV drug users)

   g. Prior to starting anti-TNF therapy

INVESTIGATIONS FOR LTBI

1. Historically, tuberculin skin tests (TST) have been available to give evidence of TB exposure. These tests have the advantage of being cheap and relatively easy to perform, but suffer from a number of problems.
2. More recently, selective immunological interferon-gamma assays (IGRAs) have been developed using the tuberculosis antigens 'early secretion antigen target 6' (ESAT-6), 'culture filtrate protein 10' (CFP-10) and tb7.7.
3. These are not present in BCG and are found in only a few species of environmental mycobacteria. Testing can be done on either cells or cell products derived from fresh blood specimens.
4. Because of the use of more specific antigens, these tests have a lower false positive rate and correlate more closely with latent infection or dormant organisms.

TUBERCULIN SKIN TESTING

1. The TST (also called the Mantoux TST) is performed by injecting a small amount of purified protein derivative from the TB bacteria (tuberculin) into the skin of the forearm. The presence of a raised, hard area or swelling is sought 48–72 hours post-injection by a trained health professional, and the reaction dimensions are measured. Redness by itself is not considered significant.
2. The interpretation of the skin test result depends on the size of the raised, hard area or swelling, as well as the person's risk of being infected with TB bacteria and the progression to TB disease if infected. The choice of cut-off points for a positive test involves trade-off between sensitivity and specificity.
3. For an initially negative test after recent exposure, screening should be repeated after 3 months as TB development may be delayed.

HOW TO INTERPRET TST SKIN REACTIONS IN THE UNITED KINGDOM

1. A TST reaction of ≥5 mm of induration is considered positive in
   a. HIV-infected persons
   b. Recent contacts of a person with infectious TB disease

c. Persons with fibrotic changes on chest radiograph consistent with prior TB

d. Organ transplant recipients

e. Persons who are immunosuppressed for other reasons

2. A TST reaction of ≥10 mm of induration is considered positive in

   a. Recent immigrants (within last 5 years) from high-prevalence countries

   b. Injection drug users

   c. Residents or employees of high-risk congregate settings (prisons, jails, long-term care facilities for the elderly, hospitals and other health care facilities, residential facilities for patients with AIDS and homeless shelters)

   d. Mycobacteriology laboratory personnel

   e. Persons with clinical conditions previously mentioned

   f. Children younger than 4 years of age

   g. Infants, children or adolescents exposed to adults at high risk for TB disease

3. A TST reaction of ≥15 mm of induration is considered positive in

   a. Persons with no known risk factors for TB

   b. Previous BCG vaccination

POSITIVE SKIN TEST

1. This indicates current or past infection with TB bacteria and additional tests are needed to determine if the person has LTBI or TB disease.

2. Only a positive TB skin test (or TB blood test) can provide information about whether a person has been infected with TB bacteria or not. It does not tell whether the person has LTBI or has progressed to TB disease. History, clinical examination and other tests, such as a chest x-ray and sputum examination, are needed to see whether the person has TB disease.

NEGATIVE SKIN TEST

1. This implies that LTBI is not likely. However, because untreated TB disease often kills, all currently available tests for LTBI are *not* considered sensitive enough to exclude active TB disease.

WHAT ARE FALSE-POSITIVE REACTIONS?

Some persons may react to the TST even though they are not infected with *Mycobacterium tuberculosis*. The causes of these false-positive reactions may include, but are not limited to, the following:

1. Infection with nontuberculosis mycobacteria
2. Previous BCG vaccination
3. Incorrect method of TST administration
4. Incorrect interpretation of reaction
5. Incorrect bottle of antigen used

WHAT ARE FALSE-NEGATIVE REACTIONS?

Some persons may not react to the TST even though they are infected with *M. tuberculosis*. The reasons for these false-negative reactions may include, but are not limited to, the following:

1. Cutaneous anergy (anergy is the inability to react to skin tests because of a weakened immune system)
2. Recent TB infection (within 8–10 weeks of exposure)
3. Very old TB infection (many years)
4. Very young age (less than 6 months old)
5. Recent live-virus vaccination (e.g. measles and smallpox)
6. Overwhelming TB disease
7. Some viral illnesses (e.g. measles and chicken pox)
8. Incorrect method of TST administration

TUBERCULIN CONVERSION

1. Tuberculin conversion is strong evidence for significant exposure to TB and is suspected when a patient with a previous negative TST develops a positive test at a later date.
2. The UK recommendation is that the two tests be done at least 6 weeks apart.

BOOSTING

1. The phenomenon of boosting can augment the response to tuberculin in repeat testing up to 2 years after the first Mantoux test.

2. When people who have had remote infection with *M. tuberculosis* and/or previous exposure to BCG are given repeated TSTs, the first test revives or primes the immune response so that with repeat testing, the response is much stronger and may lead to a false impression of conversion.

3. The UK guidelines advise two TSTs 1 week apart if boosting is suspected (e.g. in serial testing of BCG-vaccinated persons), taking the result of the second test as being the true result.

INTERFERON RELEASE GAMMA ASSAYS

TYPES OF IGRA

1. IGRAs represent a relatively new type of blood test for TB, now much more widely available. Like TST, these assays do not help differentiate LTBI from active disease.

2. There are two tests currently available:
   a. QuantiFERON®–TB Gold In-Tube test (QFT-GIT)
   b. T-SPOT®. TB test (T-Spot)

3. Both methods involve a single blood test that exploits the body's immune response to determine whether a person has been infected with TB.

4. Interferon gamma (a chemical messenger) is released by T cells that have been in previous contact with the bacterium. Stimulation is with synthetic peptides, which are specific to a small number of mycobacteria, including human *M. tuberculosis*, but not the BCG vaccine strain of *Mycobacterium bovis*.

5. Only T cells that have previously been in contact with the bacterium will release the cytokine. The amount of interferon gamma or the number of *M. tuberculosis*–sensitive T cells in the blood is then estimated by the tests.

6. IGRAs may help to avoid the costs and toxicity associated with unnecessary treatment in BCG-vaccinated individuals. In the absence of a gold standard to diagnose LTBI, the sensitivity of IGRA tests is difficult to estimate. In contact-tracing studies, they show good correlation with the degree of exposure to an index case.

7. Studies also suggest better sensitivity of the IGRA tests in particular among immunocompromised patients, among whom detection of LTBI is highly important because of the increased risk of progression to active disease.

WHAT ARE THE ADVANTAGES OF IGRAS?

1. Requires a single patient visit to conduct the test.
2. Results can be available within 24 hours.
3. Does not boost responses measured by subsequent tests.
4. Prior BCG vaccination does not cause a false-positive IGRA test result.

WHAT ARE THE DISADVANTAGES/LIMITATIONS OF IGRAS?

1. Blood samples must be processed within 8–30 hours after collection whilst white blood cells are still viable.
2. Accuracy errors in blood specimen collection or transportation.
3. Variability in assay performance and interpretation.
4. Tests may be expensive.
5. There are currently less data on the use of IGRAs for
   a. Prediction of progress to TB disease
   b. Children younger than 5 years of age
   c. Persons recently exposed to *M. tuberculosis*
   d. Immunocompromised persons
   e. Serial testing

USE OF IGRA FOR THE DIAGNOSIS OF ACTIVE TUBERCULOSIS

1. Like TST, IGRAs are basically tests for infection, and they cannot rule in or rule out active disease. Therefore, they should not be used in the first instance for the diagnosis of active TB and cannot replace appropriate microbiological and molecular investigation.
2. The UK guidelines suggest that these tests are only considered as adjunctive tools in the diagnosis of active TB if diagnosis is proving difficult and treatment options hinge upon a diagnosis (Box 8.1).

BOX 8.1: Summary of characteristics of IGRAs

- IGRAs are based on the *ex vivo* release of the key anti-MTB cytokine IFN-γ.
- IGRAs are more specific than TST and not affected by previous BCG vaccination.
- Sensitivity of IGRAs is at least equivalent to TST.
- IGRAs are similar to TST in predicting progression from latent to active TB.
- Current IGRAs are unavailable to rule in/rule out the diagnosis of active TB.
- IGRAs are increasingly incorporated into national guidelines.
- IGRAs are unable to differentiate between latent and active TB.
- IGRAs should not be used to monitor response to therapy or as a test of cure.

TST vs. IGRA

A TWO-STEP APPROACH

1. One question is whether a two-step approach should be taken or patients should have a single test, i.e. a TST or an IGRA. Provision of a standard answer to this question is difficult. Various factors influence the decision and outcome. Factors in selecting which test to use include the reason for testing, test availability and cost-effectiveness.

2. With regard to cost-effectiveness, the United Kingdom is currently adopting the two-step testing strategy in majority of the cases with a few exceptions (see later) where IGRA can be used as an alternative to TST.

3. The two-step strategy refers to an initial TST, and, if this is positive, it should be followed by an IGRA. Internationally, however, many countries have adopted a single test approach.

4. The UK guidelines recommend the following approach for different scenarios where tests for LTBI are indicated as detailed in the following (Figure 8.1).

Immunocompetent LTBI testing algorithm

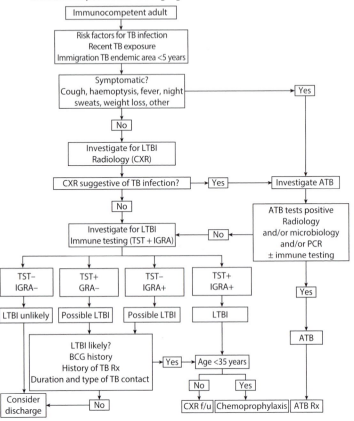

Figure 8.1 Immunocompetent LTBI testing algorithm.

CONTACT SCREENING

1. For household and non-household contacts aged >5 years
   a. Offer Mantoux testing to diagnose LTBI.
   b. Consider IGRA for individuals in whom Mantoux test is positive or for those in whom Mantoux testing may be less reliable, for example BCG-vaccinated people.
2. For household contacts aged 2–5 years

a. Offer Mantoux testing as the initial diagnostic test.
b. If the initial test is positive taking into account the BCG history, refer to a TB specialist to exclude active disease and consider treating LTBI.
c. If the initial Mantoux test is negative but the child is in contact with a person with sputum-smear-positive disease, offer an IGRA after 6 weeks and repeat the Mantoux test for increased sensitivity.
3. For household contacts aged <2 years, see the paediatric treatment chapter.
4. In an outbreak situation when large numbers of people may need to be screened, consider a single IGRA for individuals aged >5 years.

New entrants from high-incidence countries

1. Offer a Mantoux test to children aged 5–15 years. If positive, follow with an IGRA.
2. For those aged 16–35 years, offer either IGRA alone or a dual strategy.
3. For individuals aged >35 years, consider the individual risks and benefits of likely subsequent treatment before offering testing.
4. Offer Mantoux testing as the initial diagnostic test in children younger than 5 years who have recently arrived from a high-incidence country.

People who are immunocompromised

1. For people with HIV and CD4 counts less than 200 cells/mm^3, offer an IGRA and a concurrent Mantoux test. If either test is positive: perform a clinical assessment to exclude active TB and consider treating LTBI.
2. For people with HIV and CD4 counts of 200–500 cells/mm^3, offer an IGRA or an IGRA with a concurrent Mantoux test. If either test is positive, perform a clinical assessment to exclude active TB and consider treating LTBI.
3. For other immunocompromised individuals, offer IGRA alone or an IGRA with a concurrent Mantoux test. If either test is positive, perform a clinical assessment to exclude active TB and consider treating LTBI (Figure 8.2).

Immunocompromised LTBI testing algorithm

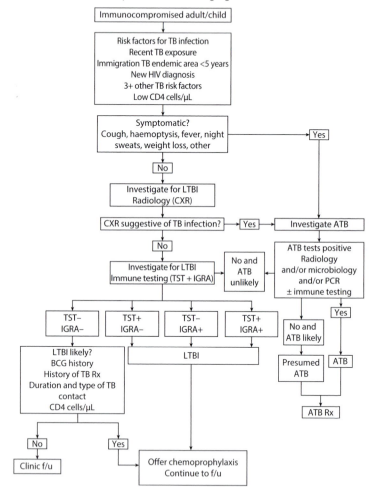

Figure 8.2 Immunocompromised LTBI testing algorithm.

HEALTHCARE WORKERS

1. For new NHS employees (not from high-incidence countries) who will be in contact with patients or clinical materials and have not had BCG vaccination, offer a Mantoux test. If the Mantoux test is negative, refer for BCG immunisation. If the Mantoux test is positive, offer IGRA.
2. For new NHS employees who have recently arrived from high-incidence countries, or who have had contact with patients in settings where TB is highly prevalent, offer IGRA.
3. For healthcare workers who are immunocompromised, these individuals should be screened in the same way as other people who are immunocompromised.

HARD-TO-REACH GROUPS

For hard-to-reach groups, offer a single IGRA.

Case study 8.2

A 40-year-old staff nurse, NB, was referred to the Occupational Health Department. His father, who lives with him, had been diagnosed with active pulmonary tuberculosis. NB did not have any particular symptoms. He smoked 10–15 cigarettes/day and consumed a moderate amount of alcohol. His past medical history included hypertension and eczema. On examination, there were no significant findings except for mild eczema. Chest x-ray was normal. Would you treat NB if he tested positive for LTBI?

TREATMENT OF LATENT TUBERCULOSIS INFECTION

RATIONALE FOR TREATMENT

1. The rationale for treating those identified by either Mantoux or IGRA to have LTBI is to kill any persisting bacilli thus reducing/preventing later reactivation of TB.

2. Treatment for LTBI can be either secondary, after LTBI has occurred (as shown by a positive Mantoux test or IGRA) or primary to try to prevent the acquisition of infection after exposure.

3. Most studies concentrate on secondary treatment for LTBI, but there are circumstances where primary treatment for LTBI may be appropriate, for example exposure of neonates to sputum-smear-positive parents or exposure of people with HIV to those with sputum-smear-positive TB.

4. An assessment of the likely benefits of treatment should be undertaken prior to commencing someone on treatment for LTBI. These should be weighed up against the individual's risk for adverse effects, and the balance is often influenced by the risk of developing TB if the LTBI is left untreated.

5. Commitment to completion of treatment and resources available to ensure adherence should also be taken into consideration. The risk/benefit profile of treatment should be discussed with the patient and the importance of adherence to therapy should be emphasised.

CURRENT UK GUIDELINES

1. UK guidelines state that once TB disease has been ruled out, treatment of LTBI should be considered for people in the following groups:

   a. People identified through screening who are 35 years or younger (because of increasing risk of hepatotoxicity with age), any age with HIV, any age and a healthcare worker and either Mantoux positive (6 mm or greater) and without prior BCG vaccination or strongly Mantoux positive (15 mm or greater), IGRA positive and with prior BCG vaccination.

   b. Children aged 1–15 years identified through opportunistic screening to be strongly Mantoux positive (15 mm or greater), and IGRA positive (if this test has been performed) and without prior BCG vaccination.

   c. People with HIV who are in close contact with people with sputum-smear-positive respiratory TB should have active disease excluded and subsequently be given treatment for LTBI.

   d. People with evidence of TB scarring on chest x-ray and an unclear history regarding completion of treatment.

2. LTBI treatment should be withheld in close contacts of people with sputum-smear-positive MDR TB who are strongly Mantoux positive (15 mm or greater), as no regimen is of proven benefit. Only a small proportion of people infected will develop the disease. Long-term monitoring should be adopted for active disease.

3. People who have agreed to receive treatment for LTBI should be commenced on one of the following regimens:
   a. Either 6 months of isoniazid (6H) or 3 months of rifampicin and isoniazid (3RH) for people aged 16–35 years not known to have HIV.
   b. Either 6 months of isoniazid (6H) or 3 months of rifampicin and isoniazid (3RH) for people older than 35 in whom treatment for latent TB infection is recommended and who are not known to have HIV.
   c. Six months of isoniazid (6H) for people of any age who have HIV.
   d. Six months of rifampicin (6R) for contacts, aged 35 or younger, of people with isoniazid-resistant TB.

4. For those declining LTBI treatment, 'inform and advise' about TB information should be given out and chest x-rays performed 3 and 12 months later to look for signs of active disease.

5. Neonates who have been in close contact with people with sputum-smear-positive TB who have not received at least 2 weeks' anti-tuberculosis therapy should be treated as follows:
   a. Neonates should be commenced on isoniazid followed by a Mantoux test after 3 months' treatment. If the Mantoux test is positive (6 mm or greater), the baby should be assessed for active TB. If this assessment is negative, then isoniazid should be continued for a total of 6 months.
   b. If the Mantoux test in a neonate is negative (less than 6 mm), it should be repeated together with an IGRA. If both are negative, then isoniazid should be stopped and a BCG vaccination performed.

6. In children older than 4 weeks but less than 2 years who have *not* had BCG vaccination and are in close contact with people with sputum-smear-positive TB, the child should be started on isoniazid and a Mantoux test performed:
   a. If the Mantoux test is positive (6 mm or greater), the child should be assessed for active TB. If active TB is ruled out, full treatment for LTBI should be given. If the Mantoux test is negative (less than 6 mm), then isoniazid should be continued for 6 weeks, followed by a repeat Mantoux test together with an IGRA.

    b. If the repeat tests are negative, isoniazid may be stopped and BCG vaccination performed. If either repeat test is positive (6 mm or greater), then the child should be assessed for active TB and consider treating for latent TB.

7. In children older than 4 weeks but less than 2 years who have had BCG vaccination and are in close contact with people with sputum-smear-positive TB, the child should have a Mantoux test:

    a. If this is positive (15 mm or greater), the child should be assessed for active TB.

    b. If active TB is excluded, then treatment for LTBI should be initiated. If the result of the test is as expected for prior BCG (less than 15 mm), it should be repeated after 6 weeks together also with an IGRA.

    c. If the repeat Mantoux test is also less than 15 mm in addition to a negative IGRA, no further action is needed. If the repeat Mantoux test becomes more strongly positive (15 mm or greater and an increase of 5 mm or more over the previous test), or the IGRA is positive, the child should be assessed for active TB.

    d. If active TB is excluded, LTBI treatment should be commenced.

8. For children requiring LTBI treatment, a regimen of either 3 months of rifampicin and isoniazid (3RH) or 6 months of isoniazid (6H) should be planned and started, unless the child is known to be HIV positive, when 6H should be given.

9. Patients in high-risk groups as mentioned earlier should be advised of the risks and symptoms of TB, on the basis of an individual risk assessment, usually in a standard letter of the type referred to as 'inform and advise' information.

RULING OUT ACTIVE TUBERCULOSIS

1. Should the results of the tests described earlier suggest that a person is infected with TB bacteria, he or she should be referred for medical evaluation to rule out TB disease. This should include a detailed medical history, physical examination, chest radiograph (x-ray) and further investigations to confirm whether the person has TB disease. A diagnosis of LTBI is made only after active TB disease has been ruled out.

2. Initiation of therapy for LTBI in patients who have active disease has significant implications in terms of promoting drug-resistant strains of TB. For this reason, it is imperative that active TB is excluded in the first instance.

SUMMARY

1. LTBI may represent previously present tuberculosis disease or current tuberculosis infection, which has not progressed to cause disease.
2. A number of risk factors have been related to progression including co-morbidity and HIV co-infection.
3. The interpretation of TST result depends on the size of the response as well as the person's risk of being infected with TB bacteria and the progression to TB disease if infected.
4. IGRAs represent a new blood test for TB, but like TST, these assays do not help differentiate LTBI from active disease.
5. Accurate contact tracing requires significant resources to identify those at risk of LTBI
6. The rationale for treating those identified by either Mantoux or IGRA to have LTBI is to kill any persisting bacilli thus reducing/preventing later reactivation of TB.

FURTHER READING

Andreu J, Cáceres J, Pallisa E, Martinez-Rodriguez M. Radiological manifestations of pulmonary tuberculosis. *Eur J Radiol* 2004 August; 51(2):139–149.

ATS (American Thoracic Society) and CDC (Centers for Disease Control and Prevention). Targeted tuberculin testing and treatment of latent tuberculosis infection. *Am J Respir Crit Care Med* 2000;161(4):221–247.

BHIVA (British HIV Association). British HIV Association guidelines for the treatment of TB/HIV coinfection. *HIV Med* 2011;12:517–524.

CDC (Centers for Disease Control and Prevention). Updated guidelines for using interferon gamma release assays to detect *Mycobacterium tuberculosis* infection. *MMWR Morb Mortal Wkly Rep* 2010;59:1–25.

Centers for Disease Control and Prevention. Tuberculosis factsheets, April 2012. http://www.cdc.gov/tb/publications/factsheets/default.htm. Accessed June 2012.

Davies PDO, Gordon GB, Davies G. *Clinical Tuberculosis*, 5th edn. CRC Press, Boca Raton, FL, 2014.

Health Protection Agency, UK. Tuberculosis general information, 2012. http://www.hpa.org.uk/Topics/InfectiousDiseases/InfectionsAZ/Tuberculosis/GeneralInformation/. Accessed June 2012.

Menzies D, Nahid P. Update in tuberculosis and nontuberculous mycobacterial disease. *Am J Respir Crit Care Med* 2013 October 15; 188(8):923–927.

National Institute for Health and Clinical Excellence, UK. Clinical diagnosis and management of tuberculosis, and measures for its prevention and control, March 2011. http://www.nice.org.uk/nicemedia/live/13422/53642/53642.pdf. Accessed June 2012.

Wrighton-Smith P, Zellweger JP. Direct costs of three models for the screening of latent tuberculosis infection. *Eur Respir J* 2006;28(1):45–50.

Tuberculosis and HIV co-infection

DANIEL KOMROWER AND MUHUNTHAN THILLAI

Case study 9.1

BL was a 36-year-old lady who reported to a local hospital with a history of severe loss of weight, fever, loss of appetite, some rashes on the body and mild cough of 3 months duration. She was treated at various clinics and hospitals without much improvement. Laboratory investigations results included a positive HIV infection but smear microscopy for TB was negative. The patient was placed on standard antiretroviral therapy (ART). Three weeks after, the patient's condition had further deteriorated. Sputum sample was taken again and sent for TB culture. The patient was started on anti-TB drugs along with modified ART while waiting for the culture result. Within a week of starting the dual therapy, the patient's clinical condition started to improve. Culture results from 4 weeks later showed tuberculous bacilli.

BACKGROUND TO HIV CO-INFECTION

1. The clinical presentation of tuberculosis (TB) has changed in countries with high human immunodeficiency syndrome (HIV) prevalence. HIV infection accelerates the natural progression of TB by diminishing cell-mediated immunity (CMI) while the immune response to TB can enhance HIV replication and disease progression.

2. The combination of these two diseases has grave implications for the already stretched public health services posing a major threat to achieving the health-related United Nations (UN) Millennium Development Goals (MDG) for TB and HIV, Stop TB Partnership's targets and universal access to comprehensive services for HIV infection prevention, treatment and care.

3. HIV is the main reason for failure to meet TB control targets in high HIV settings. HIV causes immunodeficiency and therefore increases the risk of many infections including TB.

4. TB and HIV are often referred to as the evil sisters as TB is a major cause of death among people living with HIV in sub-Saharan Africa bearing the brunt of the HIV-fuelled TB epidemic.

5. The rapidly increasing HIV epidemic in other parts of the world also increases the number of HIV-related TB cases.

EPIDEMIOLOGY OF TB AND HIV

1. TB is the cause of major morbidity and mortality globally. In 2010, WHO estimated that more than 2 billion people, a third of the world's population, were infected with tubercle bacilli with a global incidence rate of 137 cases per 100,000 population, being equivalent to about 8.8 million new TB cases annually and prevalence of 14 million.

2. It is estimated that TB kills about 1.1 million people yearly among HIV-negative people and an additional 0.35 million deaths from HIV-associated TB, 95% of these occurring in developing countries with majority in sub-Saharan Africa. Most cases were in the South-East

Asia, African and Western Pacific regions (35%, 30% and 20%, respectively) (Figure 9.1).

3. There has been steady decline in the number of HIV infections since the late 1990s with fewer AIDS-related deaths due to the scale up of antiretroviral therapy (ART).

4. Although the number of new infections has been decreasing, the relatively lower number of deaths due to HIV has resulted in an increase in the number of people living with HIV/AIDS.

5. In 2011, it was estimated that there were 2.5 million newly infected HIV patients as against 3.2 million in 2001 with an estimated 1.7 million AIDS-related deaths, which is lower than the 2.3 million in 2005. In 2011, it was estimated that 330,000 children were newly infected with HIV.

6. The burden of the disease is widely borne in the sub-Saharan Africa region where it is estimated that 70% of those infected reside. HIV infection presents as HIV I or HIV II, with the later infecting fewer people primarily in some African regions.

7. TB is the most common HIV-related complication in the world. The combined infection of TB and HIV has been christened 'the cursed duet' with both diseases creating a lethal combination and accelerating each other's progress.

8. HIV is a predisposing factor to developing active TB in individuals harbouring the mycobacterium bacilli by impairing the CMI of the patient with estimated 1.1 million patients infected with both HIV and TB globally.

9. TB is the leading cause of death among people living with HIV, with an estimated 350,000 people dying of HIV-related TB (WHO, 2011). An HIV-positive patient harbouring *Mycobacterium tuberculosis* has a 20–30 times greater risk of developing active TB compared to HIV-negative individuals. Thus, HIV infection rates in TB cases are correspondingly high in co-endemic countries such as India, China, Russia and South Africa where there is a further risk of drug-resistant TB.

10. India and China accounted for 40% of the global notified cases of TB with Africa adding another 24% in 2010. In the same year, HIV was the most important factor responsible for the increased incidence of TB in Africa. As HIV has fuelled the TB epidemic, so has TB affected significantly people living with HIV/AIDS.

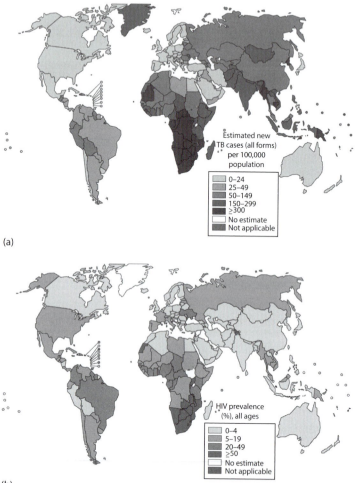

Figure 9.1 (a) Estimated global tuberculosis incidence and (b) HIV prevalence among new cases. (Reproduced from World Health Organization, Global tuberculosis report 2012, WHO, Geneva, Switzerland, 2012, available from: http://www.who.int/tb/publications/global_report/en/, cited 9 November 2012. With permission.)

NATURAL HISTORY OF TB AND HIV INFECTION

1. The natural history of *M. tuberculosis* infection indicates that the emergence of the delayed-type hypersensitivity reaction to the mycobacterium and acquired resistance are associated with the control of the initial infection in 95% of cases while 5% develop progressive TB.

2. A total of 5%–10% of the infected individuals will reactivate latent pulmonary or extra-pulmonary infections years after. It starts with individuals in close proximity to patients with TB inhaling the infectious droplet nuclei of *M. tuberculosis* from the atmosphere.

3. The inhaled bacilli reach the alveoli and are ingested by the alveoli macrophages in which they continue to replicate establishing local foci of disease called the Ghon focus. Ghon foci are transported to the hilar lymph nodes where additional foci of infection, called the primary complex, develop.

4. In most infected individuals, CMI develops 6–8 weeks after infection. T-lymphocytes are activated and together with macrophages form granulomas enclosing the bacilli and limiting its further replication and spread (Figure 9.2).

5. Many host immune cell reactions are involved in the granuloma formation. Unless a subsequent defect arises in CMI, the infection typically remains contained and active disease may never occur. This stage is usually associated with the development of a positive tuberculin skin test.

6. When the host immune response cannot contain the replication of *M. tuberculosis*, such as in HIV infection, the equilibrium formed between the host and the bacilli is disturbed and active disease occurs. HIV infection is the most important single factor in the reactivation and progression of infection in adults.

7. This occurs through dysfunctional arrays in innate immune responses that may explain why HIV-infected TB patients have accelerated course of AIDS. Blood macrophages can be infected by HIV and can thus circulate both HIV and tubercle bacilli and serve as tissue reservoir for these pathogens.

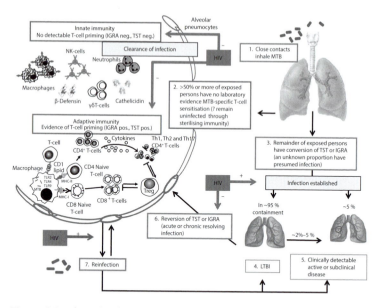

Figure 9.2 Life cycle of *M. tuberculosis* (MTB) and impact of HIV co-infection. Respirable droplets containing MTB reach the alveolar air spaces. A substantial number of individuals likely clear the infection through innate or adaptive immune mechanisms (2). These mechanisms are impaired in HIV-infected persons. The lack of T-cell sensitisation in many heavily exposed HIV-uninfected persons supports this hypothesis. A substantial remainder of exposed persons who have evidence of T-cell sensitisation (positive IGRA or TST) have presumed latent TB infection (LTBI). Only a small minority will progress in the short- or long-term to active TB (3). HIV infected persons are more likely to become infected and have a higher rate of progression from LTBI to active TB. In HIV-uninfected persons, reversion of T-cell sensitisation may signify resolving infection (6). This is likely impaired in HIV-infected persons. HIV infected persons are also more likely to become reinfected (7). (Adapted from Schwander S and Dheda K, *Am J Respir Crit Care Med*, 183, 696, 2011.)

8. The clinical presentation of TB in a patient co-infected with HIV is strongly associated with low CD4 counts, which in turn depend on the clinical stage of infection of HIV infection. TB and HIV primarily affect the CMI response. Monocytes and macrophages are important target cells for both TB and HIV and play crucial roles in their pathogenesis.

9. Infection of the macrophages with TB and HIV results in decreased cell viability, increased bacilli multiplication and altered cytokine production *in vitro*. The released cytokines thus stimulate

HIV replication. TB decreases the number of CD4 T lymphocytes. The importance of this reduction in CD4 counts is that the infected CD4 T lymphocytes are unable to control the immune response against TB and HIV.

10. Majority of TB infection occurs in the sexually active group of 15–49 years, and this is the age group when the majority of HIV infections also occur (Figure 9.3).

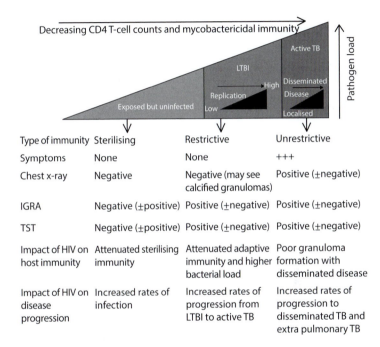

Type of immunity	Sterilising	Restrictive	Unrestrictive
Symptoms	None	None	+++
Chest x-ray	Negative	Negative (may see calcified granulomas)	Positive (±negative)
IGRA	Negative (±positive)	Positive (±negative)	Positive (±negative)
TST	Negative (±positive)	Positive (±negative)	Positive (±negative)
Impact of HIV on host immunity	Attenuated sterilising immunity	Attenuated adaptive immunity and higher bacterial load	Poor granuloma formation with disseminated disease
Impact of HIV on disease progression	Increased rates of infection	Increased rates of progression from LTBI to active TB	Increased rates of progression to disseminated TB and extra pulmonary TB

Figure 9.3 The spectrum of TB infection and the relationship between mycobacterial load and CD4 T-cell count. At one end of the spectrum are persons who become exposed but remain uninfected. These individuals likely have innate and/or adaptive immunity-related sterilising immunity. These persons are asymptomatic, and there is no radiological evidence of TB. Molecular epidemiological data support the hypothesis that HIV-infected persons are more permissive to infection. With attenuated immunity, some exposed individuals develop latent TB infection (LTBI). This occurs at a higher rate in HIV-infected persons. As CD4 counts drop, there is a higher rate of progression from latent to active TB, less well-developed granuloma formation, failure to contain the infection and, consequently, higher rates of extrapulmonary TB and disseminated disease. The pathogen load during the course of this spectrum of disease progressively increases.

FACTORS ASSOCIATED WITH INCREASED RISK OF TB AND HIV CO-INFECTION

1. Health workers are at greater risk of being co-infected with TB and HIV than most other professionals.
2. Other reported risk factors include commercial sex workers, long-haul truck drivers and poor literacy, and in some countries men are at greater risk than women.
3. Blood transfusion is also an important source of HIV infection in developing countries. Haemophiliacs and patients with sickle cell and cancer are more prone to HIV because of their regular requirements for blood and thus often dually infected with TB and HIV.
4. Drug users are prone to co-infection with TB and HIV both as a result of their communal living and sharing of infected syringes.

CLINICAL FEATURES OF PATIENTS WITH HIV AND TB INFECTION

CLINICAL PRESENTATION

1. Clinical features of patients co-infected with TB and HIV often show some variations from patients with TB alone especially in the late stages of the infection. In the early stage of infection, when the immune function is still intact, clinical feature resembles those of TB patients, with pulmonary symptoms and signs more frequently seen than extrapulmonary symptoms and signs.
2. As immunosuppression progresses, extrapulmonary TB becomes more common in patients co-infected with HIV. In patients co-infected with TB and HIV/AIDS, extrapulmonary TB is often disseminated involving, in some cases, many organs in the body.
3. There is often more generalised lymph node enlargement, more prominent in the cervical region and abdomen. Other extrapulmonary diseases commonly seen include pericarditis, peritonitis, meningitis and arthritis, and other organs in the body can also be affected. Miliary TB is more common in HIV co-infection.
4. Unlike in patients with TB infection alone, tubercle bacilli may be isolated from blood and stool culture. In the later stages of infection,

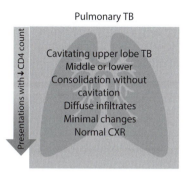

Figure 9.4 Presentation of TB in HIV-infected patients and impact of CD4 count.

cavitations are less seen but pleural and pericardial effusions are more common (Figure 9.4).

5. Patients with both infections commonly have debilitating illness with fever and weight loss more severe than in patients that are HIV negative.
6. Patients with TB should be suspected of having HIV infection where the following presentations are common:
   a. Painful generalised lymph nodes
   b. Herpes zoster (shingles)
   c. Generalised herpes simplex
   d. *Candida* infection
   e. Severe itchy dermatitis

DIAGNOSIS

1. Symptoms of TB and HIV are often similar. Patients diagnosed with TB should be counselled and tested for HIV and all patients with HIV infection should be assessed for TB.
2. The diagnosis of TB and HIV infections in a suspected patient depends on testing for both infections individually.
3. The feasibility, accuracy and operational performance of the guidelines to improve the diagnosis of TB in HIV patients by the WHO International Expert Committee were tested at different settings and found acceptable.
4. The diagnosis of TB/HIV infection involves taking a proper clinical history, physical examination, laboratory and radiographic investigations.

5. In countries with high prevalence of TB and HIV infections, the detection rate for TB is lower compared to HIV-negative TB patients owing to the paucibacillary nature of pulmonary TB in patients with HIV.

6. Patients with TB and HIV co-infection expectorate low numbers of acid-fast bacilli, and direct smear microscopy has a lower sensitivity.

7. In areas with a high HIV prevalence, WHO recommends using GeneXpert to test HIV infected individuals who have symptoms of TB, or, if not available, using culture. This approach was adopted by South Africa, but this technique should be highly developed before it can be used as the main diagnostic approach.

8. Patients co-infected with HIV and TB often present with typical radiological features different from patients with TB alone, though there might be minimal difference in the early stages of HIV infection. The spectrum of changes in chest x-ray in pulmonary TB is dependent on the relative level of immunosuppression.

9. Unlike TB infection, where most lesions are located at the apex of the lungs, patients co-infected predominantly show lower lobe disease, plural effusion, large mediastinal nodes and miliary TB.

TREATMENT

1. Treatment of TB in HIV-positive adults is generally the same as those in HIV-negative adults, with patients responding well to the 6-month antituberculosis regimen.

2. However, treatment with highly active antiretroviral therapy (HAART) for HIV infection in patients co-infected with TB frequently causes drug interaction. Patients requiring treatment are thus advised to seek care from health personnel with expertise in the management of both infections.

3. The drug/drug interactions and toxicity encountered in the treatment of patients co-infected with TB and HIV make many physicians delay HAART in patients presenting both diseases (Tables 9.1 and 9.2). However, the use of HAART in such patients has led to significant reductions in viral load and mortality.

4. WHO in its 2010 guidelines for the treatment of patients co-infected with HIV and TB recommended providing co-trimoxazole preventive therapy to all HIV-positive TB patients, when to start ART and what antiretroviral agents to use. It also recommended the 'Three I's' for

Table 9.1 Interactions between antiretroviral drugs and rifampicin and recommendations for their co-administration

Class	ARV agent	Pharmacokinetic interaction	Adjustment to ART drug dose with rifampicin
NRTIs	All	Nil	None required
NNRTIs	EFV	Mild reduction in plasma levels	None required (600 mg at night)
	NVP	Moderate reduction in plasma levels	Omit lead-in dosing and start 200 mg NVP 12 hourly
PIs	LPV/r	Significant reduction in plasma levels	Double the dose of LPV/r to 800 mg/200 mg 12 hourly[a]
	SQV/r	Significant reduction in plasma levels	400 mg SQV + 400 mg ritonavir 12 hourly[a]
	All other PIs	Significant reduction in plasma levels	Do not prescribe concomitantly
InSTI	RAL	Significant reduction in plasma levels	Double the dose of RAL to 800 mg 12 hourly

Source: Adapted from the South African HIV Clinician's Society Guidelines for Antiretroviral Therapy in Adults, 2012.

Notes: EFV, efavirenz; InSTI, integrase (strand transfer) inhibitor; LPV/r, lopinavir/ritonavir; NRTI, nucleoside reverse transcriptase inhibitor; NNRTI, non-nucleoside reverse transcriptase inhibitor; PI, protease inhibitor; RAL, raltegravir; SQV/r, saquinavir/ritonavir.

[a] Increased risk of hepatotoxicity.

reducing the burden of TB in persons living with HIV, and they include Intensified case-finding, Isoniazid preventive therapy and TB Infection control.

5. WHO recommends that all TB and co-infected patients should receive the recommended daily TB treatment during the intensive and the continuation phases and should receive the same duration of TB treatment as HIV-negative TB patients.

6. In 2009, the International Standards for Tuberculosis Care (ISTC) recommended that all co-infected HIV and TB patients receive co-trimoxazole preventive therapy and should be given throughout TB treatment. This substantially reduces mortality in HIV-positive TB patients.

Table 9.2 Adverse event profile shared between antiretroviral agents and antituberculosis drugs

Side effect	ART	Anti-TB drugs
Nausea	AZT, ddl, Pls	Pyrazinamide, ethionamide
Hepatitis	NVP, EFV, Pls	Rifampicin, isoniazid, pyrazinamide and many second-line drugs including fluoroquinolones occasionally
Peripheral neuropathy	D4T, ddl	Isoniazid, ethionamide, terizadone/cycloserine
Renal impairment	TDF	Aminoglycosides, capreomycin
Rash	NVP, EFV, RAL	Rifampicin, isoniazid, pyrazinamide, ethambutol, streptomycin and many second-line drugs including fluoroquinolones
Neuropsychiatric effects	EFV	Terizadone/cycloserine, fluoroquinolones, isoniazid

Source: Adapted from the South African HIV Clinician's Society Guidelines for Antiretroviral Therapy in Adults, 2012. With permission.
Notes: AZT, zidovudine; ddl, didanosine; Pls, protease inhibitors.

7. While ART therapy improves survival in HIV-positive patients, it also reduces TB rates of patients. ART should be initiated for *all* people living with HIV with active TB disease irrespective of CD4 cell count.
8. Mortality is high in HIV-infected TB patients despite treatment, mostly due to other complications of HIV. However, some deaths are directly due to TB infection.
9. Treatment of TB in patients co-infected with HIV greatly improves the health of such patients in most cases.

SUMMARY

1. HIV infection accelerates the natural progression of TB and has changed worldwide the presentation of the disease.
2. The burden of TB and HIV co-infection is greatest in sub-Saharan Africa.

3. Clinical presentation of TB in a patient co-infected with HIV is associated with low CD4 counts, which in turn depend on the clinical stage of infection of HIV infection.

4. Symptoms of TB and HIV can be very similar. All patients diagnosed with TB should be counselled and tested for HIV.

5. New molecular diagnostic tests such as the GeneXpert MTB/RIF assay can improve the overall sensitivity of diagnosis of TB in the setting of HIV co-infection.

6. Treatment of TB in HIV-positive adults is generally the same as those in HIV-negative adults.

FURTHER READING

Antonucci G, Girardi E, Raviglione MC, Ippolito G. Risk factors for tuberculosis in HIV-infected persons. A prospective cohort study. The Gruppo Italiano di Studio Tuberculosi e AIDS (GISTA). *JAMA* 1995;274:143–148.

Beck-Sague C, Dooley SW, Hutton MD, Otten J, Breeden A, Crawford JT, Pitchenik AE, Woodley C, Cauthen G, Jarvis WR. Hospital outbreak of multidrug-resistant *Mycobacterium tuberculosis* infections. Factors in transmission to staff and HIV-infected patients. *JAMA* 1992;268:1280–1286.

Chretien J. Tuberculosis and HIV. The cursed duet. *Bull Int Union Tuberc Lung Dis* 1990;65:25–28.

Dean GL et al. Treatment of tuberculosis in HIV-infected persons in the era of highly active antiretroviral therapy. *AIDS* 2002;16:75–83.

Global Tuberculosis Control. World Health Organization report, 2011. http://www.who.int/tb/publication/global_report/2011/gtbr11_executive_summary.pdf (accessed 09/10/12).

Golub JE, Astemborski J, Ahmed M, Cronin W, Mehta SH, Kirk GD, Vlahov D, Chaisson RE. Long-term effectiveness of diagnosing and treating latent tuberculosis infection in a cohort of HIV-infected and at-risk injection drug users. *J Acq Immune Defic Syndr* 2008;49:532–537.

Lawn SD, Churchyard G. Epidemiology of HIV-associated tuberculosis. *Curr Opin HIV AIDS* 2009;4:325–333.

Munawwar A, Singh S. AIDS associated tuberculosis: A catastrophic collision to evade the host immune system. *Tuberculosis (Edinburgh)* 2012;92:384–387.

Narain JP, Raviglione MC, Kochi A. HIV-associated tuberculosis in developing countries: Epidemiology and strategies for prevention. *Tuber Lung Dis* 1992;73:311–321.

Newman GW, Kelley TG, Gan H, Kandil O, Newman MJ, Pinkston P, Rose RM, Remold HG. Concurrent infection of human macrophages with HIV-1 and *Mycobacterium avium* results in decreased cell viability, increased *M. avium* multiplication and altered cytokine production. *J Immunol* 1993;151:2261–2272.

Patel NR, Zhu J, Tachado SD, Zhang J, Wan Z, Saukkonen J, Koziel H. HIV impairs TNF-alpha mediated macrophage apoptotic response to *Mycobacterium tuberculosis*. *J Immunol* 2007;179:6973–6980.

Pawlowski A, Jansson M, Skold M, Rottenberg ME, Kallenius G. Tuberculosis and HIV co-infection. *PLoS Pathog* 2012;8:e1002464.

Tarantino L, Giorgio A, De Stefano G, Scala V, Liorre G, Di Sarno A, Esposito F. [Diagnosis of disseminated mycobacterial infection in AIDS patients by US-guided fine needle aspiration biopsy of lymphnodes and spleen]. *Infez Med* 2004;12:27–33.

UNAIDS. UNAIDS report on the global AIDS epidemic. In: JUNPo (ed.), *HIV/AIDS*. UNAIDS, Geneva, Switzerland, 2011.

WHO. Improving the diagnosis and treatment of smear negative pulmonary and extrapulmonary tuberculosis among adults and adolescents: Recommendations for HIV-prevalent and resource-constrained settings, 2007. http://whqlibdoc.who.int/hq/2007/WHO/HTM.TB/2007.379/eng.pdf. Accessed February 1, 2015.

WHO. Global tuberculosis report 2012. WHO, Geneva, Switzerland, 2012.

Zumla A, Malon P, Henderson J, Grange JM. Impact of HIV infection on tuberculosis. *Postgrad Med J* 2000;76:259–268.

Vaccination

GARETH H JONES

Case study 10.1

AC receives a letter from the nursery that her 5-year-old son attends, informing her that a support worker who briefly worked there has been diagnosed with pulmonary tuberculosis (TB) and it is, therefore, recommended that he must be vaccinated against TB. AC is worried because her son did not receive the BCG vaccine as an infant as she was told that it wasn't routinely given in her area. However, she also has reservations because she recalls very vividly that one of her friend's foster children had become very unwell following the BCG vaccination and had nearly died, although he had subsequently suffered a lot of medical problems before being diagnosed with a weak immune system. Worried by the letter, AC tries to speak to his teacher but is informed by the headmaster that she is unavailable as she started her maternity leave the previous week. AC's parents arrive for lunch where her mother lets it be known that she doesn't think there is any point getting her son vaccinated as she recalls as a child growing up in India her two older brothers both developed consumption despite being vaccinated. However, her mother concedes that the modern vaccination may be better than the one available in the past. Her father is much more enthusiastic about BCG – he has already received half a dozen courses to treat his bladder cancer and experienced almost no side effects apart from feeling a bit fluey sometimes after a treatment and needing to pass urine more often than usual, which is annoying as he has to pour bleach down the toilet each time he goes for the entire evening on the days he has the treatment. Despite this, his urologist is very pleased with his response to the BCG treatment and intends to continue using it as ongoing therapy. Her parents leave after having a heated discussion about whether it is the same BCG that is used to treat cancer and protect against TB. AC decides to phone her sister who lives in London, who has recently qualified as a nurse, to ask her advice. Her sister seems very relaxed about BCG stating that she thinks it is very safe – as well as receiving the vaccination herself prior to starting work, all of her children have received the jab – in fact she thinks that her eldest child may have received it twice because he didn't initially develop a scar on his arm. AC's sister doesn't think her children experienced any problems after the jab, although her youngest child's scar is somewhat unsightly and she was still slightly self-conscious about it. AC is reassured but confused as to why her son wasn't offered TB vaccination whilst her sister's children were – she suspects cost may be involved as she has read many stories in the media recently about her local health authority attempting to make substantial savings by cutting services. AC spends the rest of the afternoon looking up information on the Internet where she reads about a number of exciting new vaccines being developed, some of which are about to be tested in parts of Africa. She therefore decides to make an appointment to see her general practitioner to discuss alternatives to BCG for her son.

VACCINATING AGAINST TUBERCULOSIS

PRINCIPLES OF VACCINATION

1. The general principle underpinning any type of vaccine is to invoke an antigenic response in the host immune system that induces long-term specific immunity without causing the disease itself. This is usually achieved by inoculating antigens from either the pathogen itself or an

immunologically similar organism in a non-viable state (killed or attenuated in such a way that it has a greatly reduced propensity to cause illness) during childhood.

2. It is important that any vaccination has a very low incidence of side effects given that it will potentially be administered to billions of people as well as being cheap to manufacture and easy to administer to ensure widespread uptake. The development and widespread implementation of vaccinations against infectious diseases ranks amongst man's greatest achievements.

3. The previously leading causes of disease and premature death on a global level have been controlled (MMR/polio) or eradicated completely (smallpox) by use of vaccinations. However, attempts to control TB by use of vaccination have been far less successful.

SPECIFIC ISSUES VACCINATING AGAINST MTB

1. TB is somewhat different from the other diseases that have been successfully controlled by use of vaccination; host immune response to *Mycobacterium tuberculosis* (MTB) is variable in that it may render an individual infective for a prolonged period of time and, in some cases, the pathogen is able to effectively wall itself off from the host immune system completely.

2. This means that simply pre-sensitising the host immune system by use of vaccination alone will not lead to effective disease control without concurrent identification and treatment of individuals with latent disease.

3. Bacillus Calmette–Guérin (BCG) remains the only vaccine in use today against MTB infection, and whilst it has undoubtedly impacted on the childhood burden of mycobacterial illness, it has been ineffective at controlling adult pulmonary TB; because of this as well as the growing prevalence of drug-resistant disease, the search for new vaccines continues apace.

BACILLUS CALMETTE–GUÉRIN VACCINATION

DEVELOPMENT OF BCG

1. After the successful inoculation of cowpox to protect against smallpox, attempts were made to develop a similar vaccine against TB based on *Mycobacterium bovis*. However, *M. bovis* is a virulent pathogen, and

therefore, it was not until Calmette and Guérin attenuated its pathoge-
nicity by repeatedly subculturing the organism until its virulence was
attenuated sufficiently to be used as a vaccine against MTB.

2. After over a decade of work, the resulting organism had transformed
much from the original *M. bovis* and became known as *Bacillus
Calmette–Guérin.*

STRAINS OF BCG

1. All strains of BCG available today descend directly from the original
work done by Calmette and Guérin over 100 years ago. Inevitably
once the vaccine was distributed around the world, the geographically
isolated samples underwent further molecular changes leading to the
development of genetically diverse substrains, which often were named
after the place where the receiving laboratory was situated, e.g. Montreal
and Copenhagen.

2. Therefore, although the BCG vaccine is often discussed as if it were a single entity, it should more accurately be thought of as a family of related
but subtly different substrains. To try and minimise further genetic drift
today, lyophilised reference samples are used to restock BCG supplies.

EFFICACY OF BCG

1. BCG administered to newborns has been shown to be particularly
efficacious at preventing central nervous system and disseminated
(miliary) infection by MTB in infants. Crucially important as this early
protection against these very severe forms of TB is the protective effects
induced by the vaccine wane quickly and BCG confers little protection
against pulmonary TB in adults.

2. Furthermore, BCG inoculation does do not prevent the reactivation of
latent infection. It seems that the vaccine is less effective in areas where
exposure to nontuberculous mycobacterium (NTM) is the highest
(invariably those areas with the highest burden of TB as well) as pre-
sensitisation with such antigenically similar organisms may reduce the
response to BCG itself (blocking) or the vaccine may not confer any
additional immunoprotective benefits in exposed individuals (masking).

3. Other factors influencing efficacy include co-infection with intestinal
parasites, which seem to have an immunomodulatory effect on T-cell
responses and BCG substrain used.

Cost of BCG

1. Modern vaccine can be manufactured at a very low cost with an estimated unit price of less than 0.2 USD. Maintaining a low production cost is imperative to enable continued access to the vaccine in poorer parts of the world, where the disease burden is often greatest.

Safety of BCG

1. Several billion doses of BCG have been administered worldwide since its introduction in 1921, making it the most commonly given vaccine of all time. Despite its widespread use, serious adverse reactions to the vaccine are very uncommon in immunocompetent individuals ($<1 \times 10^{-6}$).
2. Such an established safety record makes demonstrating non-inferiority of any new therapeutic agent compared to BCG very difficult.

Administration of BCG

1. Newborns should be vaccinated if they themselves or their parents or grandparents were born in an area where the annual background incidence of TB is more than 40 per 100,000 or if a direct family member has had TB in the last 5 years. This means that in some countries only certain population centres will routinely vaccinate newborns, e.g. London in the United Kingdom.
2. Older unvaccinated children up until the age of 6 with the same risk factors can also receive BCG without the need for tuberculin skin test (TST), but older children should be tested prior to vaccination. Any previously unvaccinated contact of a confirmed pulmonary TB case should also be tested with a TST prior to immunisation.
3. Unvaccinated Mantoux-negative adults under the age of 35 should be offered BCG only if they work in a high-risk occupation, especially health-care professionals with direct patient contact, including staff in non-hospital settings such as care homes or staff who are indirectly in contact with clinical specimens such as lab workers and pathologists.
4. Other professionals that are exposed to higher background rates of mycobacterium include prison workers, staff working in hostel shelters for the homeless or immigration services and any worker with exposure to animals that are reservoirs of TB-causing organisms.

5. The efficacy of vaccinating anyone over the age of 35 is unknown and therefore older unvaccinated individuals who are Mantoux negative should only be offered BCG if they are considered to be at especially high risk because of work or travel commitments.

CONTRAINDICATIONS TO BCG

1. As a live vaccine, BCG should not be administered to any individual with significant immunodeficiency, especially those infected with the human immunodeficiency virus. The use of live vaccines is also generally considered to be contraindicated during pregnancy, especially in the first trimester, and although no specific adverse effects have been reported, if deemed necessary, it is usual to delay administration of BCG until the post-partum period.

2. As with any parental therapy, anaphylaxis can occur to components of the vaccine, particularly the carrying media.

REGIMEN AND DOSE OF BCG

1. Multiple dosing schedules have not been shown to confer additional benefits compared to a once-only vaccination but does increase the likelihood of local complications.

2. BCG is usually administered as a single intradermal injection at a dose of 0.05 mL to infants under 12 months old and 0.1 mL to anyone older. A more concentrated preparation for percutaneous administration is also available which appears to be as efficacious but may be associated with a higher complication rate if accidentally injected intradermally.

3. The vaccine is injected into the top of the left arm laterally at the level of the insertion of deltoid causing a swelling to form that normally heals within a fortnight to leave a small scar. Such a uniform approach aids subsequent identification of previously vaccinated individuals and is used as a 'proof' of immunity in some circumstances.

COMPLICATIONS OF BCG

1. Hypersensitivity reactions and keloid formation are the most common early and late non-infectious complications, respectively, the latter being more common when BCG is administered above the level of insertion of the deltoid muscle onto the humerus.

2. Local infectious complications such as ulcer and abscess formation should be treated with isoniazid or erythromycin once superadded infection with other pathogens has been excluded.

3. Lymphadenopathy typically affects axillary nodes and is usually managed conservatively – chemotherapy is ineffective, so surgical management may be necessary in chronically supportive lymphadenitis.

4. Disseminated infection (BCGosis) is a rare but potentially fatal complication. The incidence is much higher in the immunocompromised and slightly higher when BCG is used as intravesicular immunotherapy due to the much higher doses administered.

5. Other systemic complications include arthritis and osteitis – the latter seemingly a strain-specific complication, being very rare outside of Scandinavia, which responds well to anti-TB agents.

INTERPRETATION OF SCREENING TESTS AFTER BCG

1. Vaccination with BCG causes cross reactivity to TSTs to develop within 2 months of administration. Generally, a higher level of induration is therefore required in previously vaccinated individuals to be considered indicative of underlying disease.

2. However, the strength of cross reactivity is variable, therefore making the interpretation of such important screening tests difficult. It is for this reason that certain low-prevalence countries (the United States, the Netherlands) have never included BCG in their national immunisation schedule.

3. Newer screening tools, such as the IGRA tests, use highly specific antigenic targets not present in BCG and, therefore, unlike tests based on tuberculin, will not give false-positive results in individuals who have been previously vaccinated.

OTHER USES OF BCG

1. Although its mechanism of action is unclear, adjuvant treatment with intravesical BCG has shown to be highly effective against recurrence of non-invasive bladder tumours that have been operatively removed. Despite the much more concentrated doses administered when used as an immunotherapy, it is still relatively rare for disseminated disease to

occur (<0.5%) and common side effects are due to direct irritation of the lower urinary tract (e.g. dysuria/frequency/haematuria).

2. Patients are reminded to pour bleach into the toilet after micturating for 6 hours following a treatment to avoid live vaccine entering the sewage system and to use barrier contraception for up to 6 weeks after their last treatment. There is currently a worldwide shortage of intravesicular BCG and it has been speculated that this will inevitably lead to higher rates of cystectomies.

3. BCG is also known to confer a level of protection against non-tuberculous mycobacterial diseases including leprosy (*Mycobacterium leprae*), Buruli ulcers (*Mycobacterium ulcerans*) and glandular diseases associated with MAC, although none of these conditions has been specifically targeted for control with the use of a vaccination programme.

FUTURE VACCINATION STRATEGIES

NEW VACCINES

The need for new vaccines against TB is clear, especially for ones effective at controlling pulmonary forms of the disease. Whilst demonstrating improved efficacy is imperative for any new vaccination, it must also be demonstrably non-inferior to BCG in terms of safety, something that may be particularly difficult with such an established record worldwide over so many years.

CLINICAL TRIALS

1. To establish clinical effectiveness and safety of new vaccines, large-scale trials must be undertaken, but with relatively low incidence of TB in most industrialised nations, often more useful information can be gathered from trails set in the third world.

2. There are however inevitably challenges in carrying out research in a resource-poor environment including a lack of regulatory bodies to provide oversight of a large-scale trail and the difficulty in obtaining truly informed consent in areas with low education and literacy levels.

3. Running a trial in a developing country means extra infrastructure costs to provide laboratory equipment and trained clinical support staff that will inevitably inflate the total budget required to bring a new

vaccine to market. As previously mentioned, carrying out trials in areas with very high background exposure to environmental mycobacterium and parasitic bowel infections may potentially confound results.

NEW APPROACHES INVOLVING BCG

1. With its established safety record and ease of administration, it is unsurprising that attempts are being made to improve the current vaccination. Now that its full genome has been established, selective genetic manipulation of BCG itself is now possible, and a number of different recombinant vaccines have been developed which could be both safer and more efficacious than the current vaccination.
2. Another line of current research looks to bolster the protective effects of BCG by involving complementary booster agents to be used alongside the current vaccine, or a recombinant version of it, to extend its protective effects into adulthood.
3. The first prime-boost candidate, MVA85A, utilises an attenuated viral vector which despite being incapable of replication is able to provoke a strong reaction from the host immune system, boosting the responses of T cells in BCG-vaccinated individuals.
4. However, in the largest trial of a new TB vaccine to date, MVA85A, although shown to be safe, did not confer any additional protection against MTB over BCG alone. Despite this set back, research continues and a variety of other immunogenic agents are being developed in the hope of extending the efficacy of BCG (Table 10.1).

NOVEL VACCINES

1. The much greater knowledge about the precise molecular components of MTB that has become available since BCG was originally introduced should mean that future vaccines are directed against much more specific antigenic targets and the way such material is presented to the immune system is also likely to change, e.g. by utilising specifically designed viral vectors administered via aerosol – a route that may be less likely to invoke anti-vector antibodies developing.
2. Whatever way vaccines are administered in future, it is also highly likely that they will include antigens expressed by MTB whilst in its dormant state, as such a strategy would potentially impact on the global

Table 10.1 Vaccine candidates evaluated in clinical trials

	Name	What is it?	Stage of testing
BCG replacements	rBCG30	Recombinant BCG expressing antigen 85B	Not in active clinical evaluation
	VPM1002	Recombinant BCG expressing listeriolysin	Phase IIa safety and immunogenicity
	Aeras 422	Recombinant BCG expressing perfringolysin and antigens 85A, B and Rv3407	Withdrawn from clinical testing
BCG booster vaccines	M72/AS01e	Fusion protein of 32 and 39 kDa antigens with adjuvant	Phase IIa safety and immunogenicity
	Hybrid I/IC31 or CAF01	Fusion protein of antigen 85B and ESAT6 with adjuvant	Phase IIa safety and immunogenicity
	HyVac IV/IC31	Fusion protein of antigen 85A and TB10.4 with adjuvant	Phase I safety and immunogenicity
	Hybrid 56/IC31	Fusion protein of antigen 85B, ESAT6 and Rv2660	Phase I safety and immunogenicity
	Aeras 402	Recombinant Ad35 expressing antigens 85A, B and TB10.4	Phase IIb efficacy
	AdHu5-85A	Recombinant AdHu5 expressing antigen 85A	Phase I safety and immunogenicity
	MVA85A	Recombinant MVA expressing antigen 85A	Phase IIb efficacy
Other whole mycobacterial vaccines	Mycobacterium vaccae	Inactivated, whole-cell M. vaccae	Phase III efficacy
	Mycobacterium indicus pranii	Heat-killed Mycobacterium indicus pranii	Phase III efficacy
	RUTI	Detoxified fragmented MTB cells	Phase IIa safety and immunogenicity

disease burden by priming the immune system to respond to the latent disease state.

3. Other preventative strategies may attempt to modulate macrophage responses to MTB either to encourage more effective clearance of the pathogen or perhaps to block uptake by phagocytes altogether, thereby preventing a latent stage or reactivation occurring.

SUMMARY

1. The only current vaccine in widespread clinical use worldwide is BCG, which has a number of drawbacks and areas of clinical uncertainty as well as several contraindications to use.
2. Novel vaccines are currently undergoing clinical trials, but to date none has shown a significant improvement on BCG.
3. The largest vaccine trial to date, MVA85A, although shown to be safe, did not confer any additional protection against MTB over BCG alone, but work is ongoing regarding a number of other vaccine candidates.

FURTHER READING

Behr MA. BCG – Different strains, different vaccines? *Lancet Infect Dis* 2002 Feb;2(2):86–92.

Behr MA, Small PA. A historical and molecular phylogeny of BCG strains. *Vaccine* 1999 Feb 26;17(7–8):915–922.

Brennan MJ, Thole J. Tuberculosis vaccines: A strategic blueprint for the next decade. *Tuberculosis* 2012 Mar;92(Suppl. 1):i, S1–S35.

Herr HW, Morales A. History of Bacillus Calmette–Guerin and bladder cancer: An immunotherapy success story. *J Urol* 2008 Jan;179(1):53–56.

Kaufmann S, Hussey G, Lambert PH. New vaccines for tuberculosis. *Lancet* 2010 Jun 12;375(9731):2110–2119.

Murphy D, Corner LAL, Gormley E. Adverse reactions to *Mycobacterium bovis* Bacille Calmette–Guérin (BCG) vaccination against tuberculosis in humans, veterinary animals and wildlife species. *Tuberculosis* 2008 Jul;88(4):344–357.

Ottenhoff THM, Kaufmann SHE. Vaccines against Tuberculosis: Where are we and where do we need to go? *PLoS Pathog* 2012 May;8(5):e1002607.

11

Tuberculosis control

MARIA ELPIDA PHITIDIS

BACKGROUND

1. Tuberculosis (TB) is arguably the world's oldest infectious disease which is still endemic. Major medical advancements have occurred over its history including establishing the use of the first stethoscope, establishing the concept of Public Health as well as founding establishments such as the Medical Research UK Council and the American Lung Association.

2. TB control is an important aspect of TB management and local, national and international guidelines exist, tailored to each institution, area or country according to its needs.

3. The primary aim of TB control is prevention. This is achieved primarily by raising TB awareness both amongst health-care professionals and amongst populations, especially when there is a high prevalence of the disease.

4. The three key objectives in controlling TB include the following:
   a. Early identification of new active disease
   b. Early, effective and completed treatment
   c. Contact tracing and notification
5. Different forms of TB control have existed throughout thousands of years, some of which have evolved to help shape current practice and help plan future policies.

HISTORICAL ATTEMPTS AT TB CONTROL

EARLY UNINTENTIONAL TB CONTROL

1. TB was originally documented in 460 BC by Hippocrates, who referred to the disease as *'phthisis'* (*Greek for* wasting of the body) [1]. He stated that it was the most common and often fatal illness of the time. Due to the high mortality, it is said that Hippocrates discouraged his physician colleagues from visiting patients with advanced disease, in order to protect their reputations.
2. This may have been the first unintentional approach to TB control, as a form of patient isolation, helping avoid transmission.

EARLY PUBLIC HEALTH

1. About 100 years later, Aristotle was the first to describe phthisis as a contagious disease. He observed that the air around the diseased is 'pernicious' and 'disease producing', and hence phthisis could be acquired by breathing that air.
2. Two millennia later, in the seventeenth century, one of the first forms of public health regarding TB arose in northern Italy, in the Republic of Lucca [2]. TB (or the so-called *consumption* at the time) became a notifiable disease.
3. In cases of fatality from consumption, by law, the belongings of the deceased had to be destroyed and doctors were obliged to perform an autopsy. The latter however was avoided by some physicians, for fear of disease transmission.

ESTABLISHING BELIEVES OF CONTAGIOUSNESS

1. In the early nineteenth century, René Laennec, arguably one of the greatest historical French physicians, invented the stethoscope. Laennec initially believed that 'phthisis is contagious only in the opinion of a few lay men and a few physicians of the South' [2].
2. He used his first stethoscope to compare his pulmonary examination findings in patients with active TB to his post-mortem findings in infected bodies and thus introduced the concept of pulmonary auscultation in diagnosing TB.
3. Coincidentally, it is believed that Laennec's stethoscope was also used by his nephew, to diagnose Laennec with the disease, who was then convinced that he had acquired this via the post-mortem studies before dying at the age of 45.

DEVELOPMENT OF SANATORIUMS

1. The first concept of a sanatorium (a medical facility for a long-term illness) was introduced by George Bodington in 1840 [3]. He wrote an essay to the President of the Council of the Central Health Board of London on the treatment of pulmonary consumption. He proposed the use of clean cool air, mild exercise, nutritious diet and convalescence, as well as the need for expert physicians who would exclusively deal with consumption in specialist centres.
2. Bodington also explained that he didn't agree with the then-mainstream treatment which he found of *utter uselessness*. This included isolation in closed rooms, *thus forcing them* (the patients) *to breathe over and over again the same foul air contaminated with diseased effluvia of their own persons*, and the use of two popular drugs, the digitalis and the tartar emetic.
3. At the time, Bodington was not received positively and articles were published against his principles in *The Lancet*. Sanatoriums however continued and spread across Europe and over the Atlantic with positive results. George Bodington was a pioneer of today's concepts of TB specialist management and infection control, but was only recognised for this after his death.

Becoming a notifiable disease and increasing awareness

1. The cornerstone in the history of TB came in 1882, when Robert Koch, a Prussian physician, identified the causal bacterium: *Mycobacterium tuberculosis* or Koch's bacillus. He verified his findings after inoculated laboratory rabbits died exhibiting symptoms of the disease.
2. The day Koch presented his findings at the Physiological Society of Berlin, the 24th of March, has been established as World Tuberculosis Day. The subsequently wider scientific acceptance of the contagious character of the disease raised the importance of TB control.
3. In 1912, TB was made a notifiable disease in the United Kingdom, and the use of sanatoria increased. Campaigns were also organised to increase awareness of the disease and to improve control, asking people to stop spitting in public places.

Establishment of tuberculosis-specific organisations

1. The Royal Victoria Dispensary for Consumption was established in the United Kingdom in 1887 [4]. Dispensaries extended their use to acting as sanatoriums for lower-income patients. The collaboration between these dispensaries and other health-care establishments became the 'Edinburgh Anti-Tuberculosis Scheme', aiming to diagnose patients at early stages of the 'dread disease'. The latter patients would be treated by the dispensaries and those with more advanced disease would be admitted to hospital in specialised wards.
2. In 1901, the 'Royal Commission Appointed to Inquire into the Relations of Human and Animal Tuberculosis' was set up. Instead of using observational studies and common believes, the commission decided to conduct experimental investigations, hence becoming a research body promoting scientific investigations. The commission developed into the UK's Medical Research Council [5].
3. Across the Atlantic, there was similar movement and the Pennsylvania Society for the prevention of TB was founded in 1892. In 1904, the National Association for the Study and Prevention of TB was founded, which then became the American Lung Association [6].

CURRENT TB CONTROL

PULMONARY TB: TRANSMISSION

1. TB transmission is airborne, which means it can be passed through the air, when a person with infectious pulmonary (or laryngeal) TB speaks, laughs, coughs or sneezes or by kissing. The larger the physical force of the activity, the more likely that this will release infected droplets into the air.
2. Smear-positive cases who have larger sputum bacillary concentrations are more infectious than only culture positive cases. The mycobacterium can stay in the air for a few hours depending on the air quality, air circulation and the presence or not of effective ventilation. If outdoors, the bacillary concentrations drop, as the infected particles tend to disperse quickly and sunlight can kill the bacilli.
3. If another person in the same area (usually in a closed room or within a short distance if outdoors) breathes in the mycobacterium, they can become infected. This can result in latent TB, a dormant stage of the infection (see Chapter 8), or active TB.
4. TB is not transmitted by shaking someone's hand, sharing food or drink, touching bed linen or toilet seats.

INFECTIOUS STAGE

1. Individuals with suspected active pulmonary TB should be treated with the same precautions as with those with confirmed active disease until proven otherwise. Confirmed infection includes smear-positive sputum for alcohol and acid-fast bacilli (AAFB) or a positive culture.
2. In both confirmed and unconfirmed cases, infection control measures should be continued, until the patient has received the first 2 weeks of combined anti-tuberculous treatment; there is evidence of smear-negative sputum and clinical improvement.
3. If not, control precautions should be continued. In cases of multidrug-resistant TB (MDR-TB), the infectious period is thought to be a lot longer and a person is only deemed non-infectious after a negative culture.

CONTROL IN HEALTH-CARE SETTINGS

1. All health-care workers should be screened for active or latent TB in pre-appointment occupational health checks. This usually involves an interview about possible exposure to TB with personal, occupational, family and travel history as well as questioning about possible symptoms which would suggest active TB infection. A review of documented evidence of BCG vaccination and of a BCG scar should also take place.

2. If such symptoms are present, urgent chest radiograph, sputum for AAFB and a referral to a respiratory physician are done.

3. A tuberculin skin test (TST) is performed to check for immunity. If this is negative, a BCG is needed (unless contraindicated). If an appropriate response is seen, as should be the case with those who are BCG vaccinated, no further actions are needed. If an exaggerated response is present, then an interferon gamma release assay (IGRA) should be done (QuantiFERON-TB or TSPOT.TB test).

4. If the IGRA is positive, a chest radiograph should be arranged and the person should be referred to a chest physician for either the treatment of latent or active TB according to the chest radiograph and bacteriology if this is needed.

5. For new staff who have recently been in areas of high TB incidence or have been in contact with patients in settings where TB is prevalent, an IGRA and a chest radiograph should be performed.

6. After the start of employment, Occupational Health should issue annual reminders to all employees about the symptoms suggestive of TB, as well how to report these.

7. Administrative control aims to reduce infection risk in a larger group of people [7]. Health-care institutions, especially those that are likely to treat patients with active TB, should have readily accessible guidelines about what to do when this is suspected. The TB infection control strategy should give equal weight, firstly, on the early identification of the disease, secondly, on preventing transmission and, thirdly, on treating it. Furthermore, there should be a dedicated staff member with specialist knowledge and experience who can be contacted for advice.

8. Single side rooms should be used for such patients with the doors closed at all times. Clear signage should exist outside these rooms, to ensure both staff and visitors are informed of the necessary infection control

precautions in place. No contact with other patients should be allowed. Unnecessary transport within the hospital should be avoided, minimising the number of areas which can be exposed to the mycobacterium. If a transfer is necessary, the patient should wear a protective surgical mask. Strategies should also exist to alert the ordering physician, if a TB test is positive. Education and training also plays a large part in TB awareness and control.

9. Environmental control aims to reduce the ambient room air concentration of the mycobacterium, preventing spread. Effective ventilation removes contaminated air from the room and replaces it with air free of mycobacteria from outside air, air from a low-risk area in the building or recirculated air which has been treated to kill or remove the bacilli. The air-flow direction is important to ensure that the clean air completely mixes with ambient room air and outflow air is removed away from other patient areas, windows and ventilation inlets.

10. Air filtering occurs through the use of high-efficacy particulate air filtration or ultraviolet germicidal irradiation. Air filtration though is not a substitute of good ventilation. Use of respiratory protective equipment aims to reduce the risk of exposure to health-care workers. When high-risk exposure is predicted, respiratory protective equipment should be used. High-risk exposure happens with cough-inducing procedures such as nebulised medications and the use of ventilators, or if undertaking an endoscopy. This is also the case when entering a patient's side room, as higher concentrations of infected air particles are predicted.

11. The Occupational Health and Safety Departments should ensure that all health-care professionals who could be involved with the management of such patients should have training and fit testing of specialised masks, which are mechanical filter respirators with an exhalation valve. The respirators should be up to FFP3 or N95 standard and are available in different sizes, to ensure best fit, aiming for a less than 10% seal leakage.

12. Other personal protective equipment such as aprons and gloves are commonly used by all staff when entering a patient's side room as part of standard contact precautions. Other equipment such as gowns and eye protection must be risk assessed as necessary by individual staff, depending on the risk of coming into contact with infected bodily fluids, including sputum.

13. Medical equipment used with TB patients should ideally be of single use, or single patient use. If this is not possible, equipment should be cleaned and sterilised before their removal from the room. Furthermore, patients with TB or suspected TB should be the last ones on lists for endoscopy or other procedures, in order to minimise potential transmission to other patients.

14. Only close household contacts should be permitted until a patient is deemed non-infectious. Other contacts should be allowed only at the discretion of the staff. Visitors in general should be advised to report to the nurse in charge on arrival, wash their hands when entering and leaving the room and not to visit other patients on the ward. Furthermore, visitors should not bring children along who have not received their BCG vaccination.

15. When a patient is deceased, a body bag should always be used for both confirmed and suspected cases of both pulmonary and extrapulmonary TB. This should be labelled as 'danger of infection' in order to protect mortuary and pathology staff.

MULTIDRUG-RESISTANT TB AND SPECIAL PRECAUTIONS

1. When MDR-TB is suspected, the following precautions are required:
   a. Rapid diagnostic tests for resistance.
   b. Prompt initiation of treatment and effective infection control should be started, even if results are awaited.
   c. Transfer the patient to a negative pressure room. If such facilities are not present, the patient should be transferred to another hospital, where negative pressure side rooms and medical expertise in treating MDR-TB exist.
   d. Staff and visitors should wear a respirator mask to FFP3 standard during any patient contact.

TB CONTROL IN THE COMMUNITY

1. If a patient is being treated in the community, similar infection control precautions exist. Those with active infectious TB should not go to work or school and avoid being in enclosed areas where they might be a risk

to others, as well as try and avoid contact with children, until they are deemed non-infectious after discussion with a specialist.

2. It is advised that during the infective stage, they wear surgical masks to minimise potential transmission to others and leave windows open if not too cold to allow air circulation, which leads to lower concentration of infected air particles. If they are expectorating, this should be done by covering their nose and mouth with a paper handkerchief (or other equivalent) and disposing this appropriately in a plastic bag.

3. Regular hand washing should also be recommended. Clothes, linen and cutlery should be washed as normal at home, on a regular basis. After the initial infective period has ended, people can go back to their daily routines.

4. Both in hospitals/other health-care institutions and in community, each patient should be allocated a TB specialist nurse. She or he will follow the TB cases up, ensuring the completion of appropriate treatment, monitoring for side effects of the latter and providing support when needed. TB specialist nurses are usually also the ones responsible for arranging contact tracing and their screening.

CONTACT TRACING

1. Contact tracing aims the following:
   a. To reduce further TB-associated morbidity and mortality by detecting and treating either latent or early active disease.
   b. To stop further TB transmission, by treating contacts that could have otherwise become infectious themselves.
   c. This should be done as soon as possible after the confirmation of pulmonary TB in the index case.

2. The likelihood of infection and degree of contact tracing depend on the following factors:
   a. The index case's infectiousness.
   b. How long they are likely to have been infectious for. It is difficult to establish the onset of infectiousness. This is considered to be the time of onset of cough. If there is no cough, then the onset is that of the first TB-related pulmonary symptom. If the onset of the disease remains unclear, then for screening purposes, contacts are traced if they have been in contact with the index case in the 3 months prior to the diagnosis.

    c. The length of exposure. The arbitrary cumulative number of hours for significant exposure of non-household contacts is 8 if smear positive and 40 if only culture positive.

    d. Place of exposure. Determines the bacillary air concentration and hence likelihood of transmission.

    e. The characteristics of the contact, e.g. age and immune status.

3. Every case of confirmed pulmonary TB should be interviewed promptly in order to identify a possible source and possible contacts at risk. The interview should be in two parts.

    a. The first should establish how long the index case has been infectiousness for.

    b. The second should include the index case's daily routine and household contacts, recent high-risk proceedings like respiratory, otorhinolaryngological and dental procedures triggering respiratory manoeuvres like coughing, occupational history including contact with colleagues and travel history including any recent long-haul flights in the preceding 3 months.

4. Contacts are prioritised for screening into high-, medium- and low-priority risk groups. High-risk contacts are screened first, followed by those of medium and then low risk. If however the higher-priority contacts do not show any evidence of transmission, lower-risk groups might not be screened.

5. In cases of time delay in the diagnosis of a smear-positive index, screening of medium-risk groups could be considered before the investigations for the high-risk group are complete. Low-priority contacts are only screened after a 6–8-week follow-up and only if there is evidence of transmission in the higher groups.

6. High-risk contacts include those with the most significant exposure, usually household contacts, as well as those who are at higher risk of developing active disease from transmission. The latter group includes young children and those with immunosuppression, either through HIV or other immunosuppressive conditions and medications, as well as those who are malnourished or have conditions that predispose them to hypoproteinaemia.

7. Even though infection with MDR-TB is associated with increased mortality and morbidity, there is no evidence to suggest that its mode of transmission is different to drug-sensitive TB or that contact tracing is done in a different way.

NOTIFICATION

1. When a doctor confirms or is highly suspicious that a patient has TB, he or she is then responsible for immediately informing the appropriate local authority, or the Consultant of Communicable Diseases stating the following:
   a. Name, age and sex of the patient
   b. Patient's current address (including hospital's address if so)
   c. Condition, i.e. TB and the likely onset
   d. Date of admission to hospital (Figures 11.1 and 11.2)

TRAVEL

1. Travellers should avoid spending a lot of time in high-risk enclosed areas (i.e. hospitals, shelters) especially in high-risk countries. Those who travel to work in such areas should enquire about the local

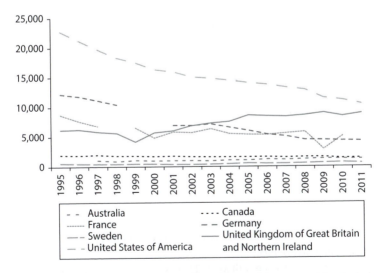

Figure 11.1 TB notification rates in selected low-incidence countries, including the United States, Australia, Canada, the United Kingdom, Germany, France and Sweden between 1995 and 2011. (From World Health Organization, Global tuberculosis report 2012, WHO, Geneva, Switzerland, 2012.)

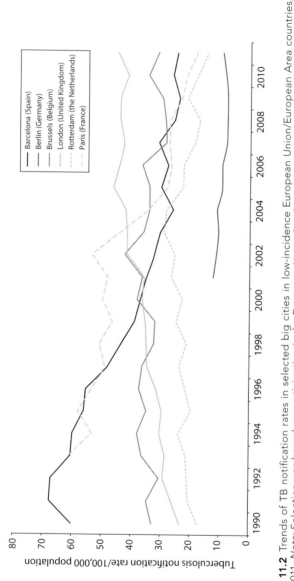
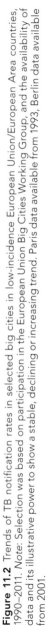

Figure 11.2 Trends of TB notification rates in selected big cities in low-incidence European Union/European Area countries, 1990–2011. Note: Selection was based on participation in the European Union Big Cities Working Group, and the availability of data and its illustrative power to show a stable, declining or increasing trend. Paris data available from 1993, Berlin data available from 2001.

workplace policies for TB infection control, including the use of protective respirators. It is advisable that on return to their country of origin, the workers should be re-screened for TB.

2. For immigration purposes, different countries have different rules for immigrants from high-risk countries, including people with short-term work visas or those requiring a visa for a period of more than 3 months, refugees, asylum seekers and students, amongst other groups.

3. Some countries require TB screening in the country of origin, and in such cases, a person could become infectious between the time of screening and arrival to the host country. Other countries require screening on entry to the country. Some countries on the other hand require both screening in the country of origin and on arrival.

4. The rising number of air passengers makes it difficult to screen everybody for TB, and hence only those who travel for immigration purposes get screened.

5. If a passenger has TB, the risk of transmission depends on the severity of the disease, the time length of the flight (long-haul flights of more than 8 hours pose greater risk) and the cabin's air quality. The 2008 WHO guidelines on tuberculosis and air travel [8], however, state that no case of clinically or bacteriologically confirmed TB disease has been identified as a result of air travel–related exposure during flight. In general, less than 10% of those with latent TB will develop the active disease during their lives and this can develop after many years. Considering this, therefore, the possibility of acquiring active disease in the future due to air travel cannot be excluded.

6. Airlines are obliged to comply with the laws of the countries in which they operate. They are also obliged to inform the relevant health authority if they suspect or know that a passenger or crew member has a notifiable disease such as TB. This does not break confidentiality rules, as it is done for public health purposes. The same applies when a list of passengers and crew is provided to the public health services for contact tracing and notification.

7. Air travel is not allowed if a person is known to have infectious TB and boarding can be refused in such a case. Furthermore, the WHO guidelines on air travel state that if a physician knows that a person with infectious TB is planning to travel on a commercial airline against medical advice, the public health authority should be informed in

writing. Once patients with drug-sensitive TB are deemed non-infective (usually after 2 weeks of treatment and a good clinical response), they are allowed to travel. In cases of MDR-TB, patients cannot travel until they are proven non-infective with negative cultures.

8. In cases when a person with infectious TB needs to travel, this should be done by alternate means, such as air ambulances, ground transportation or private carriers.

9. If a passenger develops symptoms suggestive of TB whilst on a flight, the crew should try to relocate that person if possible in an area where there are not many others in close proximity. That person should be given a surgical face mask or paper towels for application in front of his/her mouth and nose when talking or coughing, to prevent potential spread. A designated crew member only should look after that person, who should be taking the same precautions (i.e. wearing gloves) as when dealing with any other potential infectious material, and wear protective equipment such as a face mask (if this not tolerated by the person who is exhibiting symptoms). The pilot should inform air traffic control of the above possibility, who will then inform the local public health authority.

10. When a new case of active TB is identified, a travel history should be taken. If there is a history of a long-haul flight (more than 8 hours) in the preceding 3 months, public health authorities should be appropriately notified. If needed, the authorities liaise with the airline for contact tracing of the passengers in the same row and two rows ahead and behind of the TB case. If the TB case is a crew member, passengers are not deemed close contacts, due to limited exposure. Work colleagues, however, with high exposure risk would be screened instead. The public health authorities at the country of destination liaise with the corresponding authorities at the country of origin to coordinate their efforts.

LATENT TB

No infection control is required unless this reactivates. However, if a group of related cases with latent TB is found, then an attempt to find the potential source should be made. Examples of related cases include close contacts, such as from the same household, school or workplace.

Extrapulmonary TB

No infection control is required, unless there is an open wound containing the mycobacterium. If so, standard protective equipment should be worn. However, investigations should take place (chest radiograph, induced sputum or bronchioalveolar lavage) to ensure there is no concurrent pulmonary disease.

WORLDWIDE TB CONTROL

Directly observed treatment short course

1. Directly observed treatment short course (DOTS) is an internationally recommended WHO strategy for TB control, which was introduced in the mid-1990s. It has been recognised as a highly efficient and cost-effective strategy of five components:
   a. Sustained political and financial commitment
   b. Diagnosis by quality-assured bacteriology
   c. Standardised short-course anti-TB treatment, given under direct and supportive observation
   d. Regular uninterrupted supply of high-quality anti-TB medications
   e. Standardised recording and reporting
2. DOTS-Plus was developed in 1998 to include MDR-TB. It requires the capacity to perform tests for drug resistance, which is not routinely and universally available, as well as the availability of MDR-TB treatment. Monthly surveillance until cultures show negative results is recommended for DOTS-Plus, but not for DOTS [9,10].

Stop TB partnership

1. An unplanned TB Epidemic Committee met in London in 1998 after the rise in global TB epidemic, and the first Stop TB Initiative was established. In 2000, this produced the Amsterdam Declaration to stop TB, calling for action from the top 20 countries in terms of TB burden. On the same year, the Health Assembly of the WHO sanctioned the Global Partnership to Stop TB [11].
2. Currently the 'Stop TB Partnership' involves nearly 1000 organisations, working together to improve the following seven areas: DOTS

expansion, TB/HIV, MDR-TB, new TB drugs, vaccines, diagnostics and a global laboratory initiative. The partnership's targets aim to reduce TB prevalence and death rates by 50%, compared with their levels in 1990 and to reduce the global incidence of active TB cases to <1 case per 1 million population per year by 2050.

FUTURE OF TB CONTROL

1. The primary aim of current and future TB control is to successfully stop its transmission via early identification and treatment of the disease. The current reporting system needs to improve as globally one in three estimated cases of TB is not reported or does not reach health-care services.
2. TB awareness must be raised, not only amongst populations but also amongst local and international organisations, governments, charitable and profitable medical establishments. All should work together in order to achieve the most optimum TB control possible, ensuring that TB cases are reported correctly and only once if a TB case moves from one area or establishment to another.
3. The WHO together with the Stop TB strategy and civil society organisations will continue to work closely together and try to eliminate TB.

STOP TB STRATEGY

1. The Stop TB strategy [10,11,12], established in 2006, was designed by the WHO and the Stop TB Partnership as an extension to DOTS and is based on the United Nations Millennium Development Goals (MDGs). These were established as a guideline for international cooperation aiming to reduce poverty and improve health. TB is one of the MDG's priorities aiming to reduce its incidence.
2. The Stop TB Strategy's vision is a world free of TB. It builds on current achievements and is in accordance with the 2005 World Health Assembly resolution on sustainable financing for TB control. Its six basic components are as follows:
   a. Pursue high-quality DOTS expansion with continuous monitoring and evaluation.
   b. Address TB/HIV, MDR-TB, by collaborating with other organisations and by reaching vulnerable groups.

   c. Contribute to health system strengthening, by improving human resources, financing, management, service delivery and information systems.

   d. Involve all care providers, by using public–public and public–private mix approaches, including the International Pharmaceutical Federation.

   e. Empower communities and people with TB by means of advocacy, communication, social mobilisation and community-based TB care.

   f. Enable and promote medical and operational research.

3. In a 15-year period between 1995 and 2010, 55 million patients were treated for TB under the DOTS/Stop TB Strategy. Of these, 46 million were successfully treated, saving an estimated 6.8 million lives when compared to the pre-DOTS standard of care.

CIVIL SOCIETY ORGANISATIONS

1. These are 'third sector' non-profit, non-governmental, community- and patient-based organisations and professional associations whose aim is to promote the well-being of the communities they represent [13,14]. (First and second sectors are the government and private-for-profit organisations.) Their role is vital, especially in the poorer and most remote and vulnerable areas when they provide medical care and general support when other institutions cannot reach the patient.

2. Civil society organisations also aid research, manage charitable funds and promote community development, whilst engaging in health promotion and welfare support. They understand the local circumstances and thus are invaluable advocates in coordinating discussions between the locals and the government.

3. The WHO encourages the work of civil society organisations for controlling, managing and preventing TB worldwide. Its Stop TB Department met a selected group of civil societies in October 2010 in Geneva to find ways of strengthening their role. They agreed that the WHO and its partners should utilise TB ambassadors to encourage and facilitate these organisations and agreed to help with training and technical support and with linking them to the Global Fund authorities. Furthermore, they concluded that the WHO would include civil society organisations in its global TB policy and decision-making bodies. The WHO will also promote further meetings in the future amongst

key-role players in TB, aiming to develop global-, regional- or country-specific roadmaps, engaging civil society organisations in TB prevention, care and control.

4. By enhancing the role of these organisations in the future, they will be more able to liaise with local medical and political authorities, ministries, United Nations agencies and pharmaceutical and charitable organisations, amongst others. The aim is to help transform local, national and global responses to TB.

SUMMARY

1. TB has been present for many thousand years, but it was only after the discovery of mycobacteria as the causative organism in the late nineteenth century, that public health control measures came into force including the labelling of TB as a notifiable disease and the development of sanatoria.
2. TB control is under the care of both national and international organisations which aim to promote awareness, prevention, treatment and infection control.
3. Contact tracing is an important part of TB control and should be carried out in a systematic manner.
4. Health-care institutions should have their own methods of TB control and containment to prevent the spread of disease either to health-care workers or to non-infected patients.
5. Strategies including DOTS and Stop TB have been used in recent years to try to stop the spread of TB.

REFERENCES

1. Herzog, H. History of tuberculosis. *Respiration* 1998;65:5–15.
2. Sepkowitz, K.A. Tuberculosis and the health care worker: A historical perspective. *Ann Int Med* January 1994;120:71–79.
3. Keers, R.Y. Two forgotten pioneers: James Carson and George Bodington. Thorax 1980;35:483–489.
4. The Edinburgh anti-tuberculosis scheme. *Br J Nurs* February 1914:177.
5. Medical Research Council, About. http://www.mrc.ac.uk/about/history/. Accessed on 4 November 2015.

6. American Lung Association, Mission Impact and History. http://www. lung.org/about-us/our-history/. Accessed on 4 November 2015.

7. Infection Control in Health-Care Settings Fact sheet; Centres for Disease Control and Prevention, May 2012.

8. WHO. *Tuberculosis and Air Travel: Guidelines for Prevention and Control*, 3rd edn., 2008.

9. Global Tuberculosis Control, WHO report 2011.

10. The Stop TB Strategy: Building on and enhancing DOTS to meet the TB-related Millennium Development Goals. TB Partnership, WHO 2006.

11. Stop TB Partnership. http://www.stoptb.org/. Accessed on 4 November 2015.

12. *Implementing the Stop TB Strategy: A Handbook for National Tuberculosis Control Programmes*, WHO, Geneva, Switzerland, 2008.

13. Report of a WHO consultation on strengthening the active engagement of civil society organizations in the global TB prevention, care and control efforts. Geneva, Switzerland, September 30–October 1, 2010.

14. Transforming the global TB response through effective engagement of civil society organisations: The role of the WHO. Bulletin of WHO, 2011.

FURTHER READING

Bhutta ZA, Lassi ZS, Pariyo G, Huicho L. Global experience of community health workers for delivery of health related millennium development goals: A systematic review, country case studies, and recommendations for integration into National Health Systems. Global Health Workforce Alliance and World Health Organization, Geneva, Switzerland, 2010.

Chowdhury AMR et al. Control of tuberculosis by community health workers in Bangladesh. *Lancet* 1997;350:169–172.

de Vries G et al.; the Tuberculosis in European Union Big Cities Working Group. Epidemiology of tuberculosis in big cities of the European Union and European Economic Area countries. *Euro Surveill.* 2014; 19(9):pii:20726.

Haileyesus G, Thomas J, Tomaskovic L, Raviglione M. Engage-TB: Integrating community-based tuberculosis activities into the work of nongovernmental and other civil society organizations: Operational guidance. World Health Organization, Geneva, Switzerland, 2012.

Mookherji S, Weil D. Food support to tuberculosis patients under DOTS: A case study of the collaboration between the World Food Program and the National TB Control Program in Cambodia, December 8–17, 2002. Management Sciences for Health and Stop TB Partnership, Arlington, VA, 2005.

Obermeyer Z, Abbott-Klafter J, Murray CJ. Has the DOTS strategy improved case finding or treatment success? An empirical assessment. *PLoS One* 2008;3(3):e1721.

World Health Organization. Community contribution to TB care: Practice and policy. Review of experience of community contribution to TB care and recommendations to National TB Programmes. Stop TB Department, WHO, Geneva, Switzerland, 2003.

World Health Organization (WHO). Global tuberculosis report 2012. WHO, Geneva, Switzerland, 2012.

Zumla A, Grange JM. Doing something about tuberculosis. *Br Med J* 1999;318:956.

Index